Doulas and Intimate Labour

Doulas and Intimate Labour

Boundaries, Bodies, and Birth

EDITED BY

Angela N. Castañeda and Julie Johnson Searcy

DEMETER

DEMETER PRESS, BRADFORD, ONTARIO

Funded by the Government of Canada
Financé par la gouvernement du Canada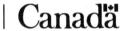

Demeter Press
140 Holland Street West
P. O. Box 13022
Bradford, ON L3Z 2Y5
Tel: (905) 775-9089
Email: info@demeterpress.org
Website: www.demeterpress.org

Demeter Press logo based on the sculpture "Demeter" by Maria-Luise Bodirsky <www.keramik-atelier.bodirsky.de>

Front cover artwork: Amanda Greavette, "Love is All" (Love is all you need, all you need is love," Lennon/McCartney), 2011, oil on canvas, 4.5 x 3.5 feet. Website: amandagreavette.com.

Printed and Bound in Canada

Library and Archives Canada Cataloguing in Publication

     Doulas and intimate labour : boundaries, bodies, and birth / editors, Angela N. Castañeda and Julie Johnson Searcy.

Includes bibliographical references.
ISBN 978-1-926452-13-5 (paperback)

     1. Doulas. 2. Mothers. 3. Childbirth. I. Castañeda, Angela N., 1976-, author, editor II. Searcy, Julie Johnson, 1979-, author, editor

RG950.D69 2015   362.1982   C2015-908173-4

The way a culture treats women in birth is a good indicator of how well women and their contributions to society are valued and honored.

—Ina May Gaskin

Table of Contents

Acknowledgements

This book is about the complex relationships surrounding reproduction and birth. The voices that shape this volume offer us access to intimate moments. We are first and foremost indebted to the women, families, and birth workers who graciously shared their lives with us.

Our gratitude also extends to Demeter Press and Dr. Andrea O'Reilly for embracing the idea for this volume. Heartfelt thanks go to Amanda Greavette, whose stunning cover art for this book beautifully captures the intimacy of birth. And to all of the contributors who joined us on this journey, we are grateful for your energy and expertise and are honoured to have worked with you on this project.

We are also thankful for institutional support from both DePauw University and Indiana University. Our deepest thanks extend to the many colleagues and friends at both universities and in our community who provided motivation and support for this project. And to the special circle of women that surround us, we thank you for being present for us throughout this process.

Finally, we are grateful to our families, especially our parents, Hank and Rochelle Martin, and Brad and Rosie Johnson, whose love and encouragement are behind our every word. And to our husbands, Ernesto and John, who took care of kids when we had to travel to conferences or to work late writing, and who nourish us with their infinite love, patience, and unwavering support. And lastly, to our children, Joyce, Max, Grace, Eloisa, Sam, and James—you are our inspiration, joy, and strength.

Foreword

ROBBIE DAVIS-FLOYD

"TO DOULA OR NOT TO DOULA?" That is the question this cogent and timely book answers with a resounding, "To doula!"

First of all, after reading the introduction, I was personally both astonished and intrigued by the many kinds of doulas in practice and the depth and variety of the kinds of care they provide for a wide range of mothers. Evidently, the full spectrum of doula care includes not only pregnancy, labour/birth and postpartum care, but also care for women experiencing abortions, adoption, birth during incarceration, and baby injuries or anomalies and deaths. I learned from other chapters that there are also hospice doulas, doulas who specialize in caring for teens or military personnel, "radical" doulas, hospital-based doulas, and homebirth doulas.

One of the great strengths of this book is that most of its chapters are written by women who have practised as doulas or are practising doulas themselves. Thus, they are able to write "from the inside," in what anthropologists call an "experience-near" manner that draws the reader in because of the ways in which the authors sometimes incorporate their personal experiences (both of being a doula and of receiving doula care) into their narrations, bringing a strong sense of vitality and immediacy to the anthropological studies they present.

If you want to know why doulas matter, read chapter one by Megan Davidson on how doulas improve birth outcomes—it provides a succinct summation of the proven benefits of doula care. Davidson enlivens the data through ethnographic accounts taken from her interviews with experienced doulas, who have much to say about *why* the well-known *doula effect*—that is, the fact that doula care improves both the physiological and the psychological outcomes of birth—is real and so very potent for the mothers receiving that care. Davidson manages to present a countervailing argument to Norman and Rothman's widely known suggestion that rather than making birth better for women, doulas just make women feel better about bad births. Davidson's interviewees stressed "intimate connection and individualized decision-making" as two of the primary reasons for the doula effect. The intimate connection comes from many hours spent together with the mom before labour starts, getting to know her and her needs and desires, resulting in the doula's ability to help the mother make individualized decisions about action and treatment during labour and birth.

The continuity of doula care—the fact that to produce the doula effect, the doula must be consistently present with the mother throughout the labour and birth—is stressed in this chapter and throughout this volume, as well it should be. I have my own quirky theory about why the doula effect only occurs if the doula is continuously present. I have always felt (and experienced in my own two births with doulas at my side) that a web of energy forms between the mom and the doula during labour, and it's a fragile one—it can be easily disrupted by the doula's absence from the mother's side for more than a few minutes at a time. To me, it seems that maintaining this web of energy is the doula's primary job, because within that energy field, the mother and the doula can establish a strong psychic bond, enabling the doula's positive energy field to help the mother maintain her own positive energy during her labour travails.

This quirky little theory of mine is based on my understanding of what I have long called "the holistic model of medicine" (Davis-Floyd "Models of Birth"; Davis-Floyd *Birth as an American Rite of Passage*): a paradigm of care based on the notion that the body is an energy field in constant interaction with other energy fields; thus negative energy at a birth (say from an unkind hospital attendant or an overanxious mother-in-law) can negatively affect the birth process, while positive energy can help that process flow smoothly. As I have often stated in my talks all over the world, *if you intervene at the level of energy, you don't have to intervene at the level of technology.* The doula can politely ask the anxious mother-in-law to leave the room. She can become a tactful buffer between the unkind nurse and the vulnerable labouring mom. If labour stalls, she can ask the mother if she is afraid of anything, and then help her express and release any fears that might be impeding her labour.

Good, experienced doulas, to my way of thinking, are experts at detecting and getting rid of negative energy during labour and replacing it with the positive energy that can get the labour process back on track. They might get the mother up to dance to a happy rock n' roll song, or throw open the window shades to let in the sunlight, or tell a joke to get everyone laughing, or get a mother to change any tight, high squeaky sounds that she might be making to low, deep guttural sounds that open her throat. Why? Because, responds the holistic midwife or doula, there is an energetic connection between the throat and the cervix: if the throat is closed up tight from anxiety, tension, or fear, then the cervix will be too. Opening the throat opens the cervix. So the doula might help the mother do that by making low, deep guttural sounds and by modelling them for the mother until she picks up those sounds and begins making them herself—something she might have been too embarrassed to do on her own. She and the doula can achieve *rhythmic entrainment* (Davis-Floyd and Laughlin *The Power of Ritual*) when they chant together and, synchronistically, the hormones flow.

In chapter two, Alison Bastien unpacks the magic of doula care. Her apt metaphors include helping the mother to "map" not only the outer cultural "journey"—the "signposts" of which include prenatal exams and testing, choosing the place of birth, epidurals and inductions, the process of cervical dilation, cloth diapers or disposable ones, and so on—but also the inner journey. Noting that doulas can get in the way of that inner journey, Bastien cites research on the brainwave states that the mother moves through during labour and birth—beta, alpha, theta, and delta (the deep unconscious). She describes how she draws maps on a board for an upriver trip in a kayak—a lovely metaphor for the labour-birth process. As the strong current draws the mother's kayak away from her companions, she passes through the four brain states (which Bastien brilliantly corresponds with stages of cervical dilation) and finally enters that deep delta state in which she lets the waterfall take her until she reaches a still, calm pool where her body does its work to birth the baby while the mind stays out of the way. When the woman is in that state, it is the doula's job, Bastien recommends, to let go of "cheerleading" and to stay out of the way, too.

Michel Odent calls this state "going to another planet"; I experienced it as going deep down inside myself to a place no one else could touch, where there was only me and the pain—and suddenly, I went over the waterfall and gave myself up to the pain. In that full surrender, there was no more separation between me and the pain. I became the pain. We were one. And in that oneness, I experienced a bliss so profound that its feeling has stayed with me to this day. My two midwives and one doula (now my best friend) followed Bastien's recommendations: they simply left me alone in that still, deep pool until the need to push brought me up and out of it and led to the wondrous home birth of my son. Floating in that deep pool (I personally experienced it as floating some feet above my body) in that profound state of oneness and bliss enabled me to find the energy that I needed to push out my ten-pound baby after a pretty exhausting three-day labour.

Bastien is right. Sometimes doulas do need to just get out of the way (and keep others away, too) and let the mother stay in that deep delta state for as long as she needs. In such instances, as Bastien describes, the doula doesn't have the map but rather follows the mother as she journeys into her place of stillness, surrender, and power. She concludes her magical chapter thus: "This is the skill I would challenge the doula to hone—not her knowledge, her tricks, her passion, her outrage, nor her love—but her willingness to share the map inward and let the woman go."

In chapter three, Sarah Lewin gives us a whole new set of understandings regarding why doulas matter, in ways that I personally had never previously considered. She's all about body politics and how our cultural *supervaluation* (Davis-Floyd 2004) of thinness in women negatively affects mothers and doulas alike. Noting that "doulas and birth advocates support the belief that birth is an opportunity for women to reclaim their bodies," she goes on to show how doulas can help women rewrite their body narratives in a new language of power and embodied wisdom. And as doulas do so, they can help themselves to accomplish the same.

In chapter four, Susanna Snyder examines the amazing ways in which doulas can empower birth mothers who choose to give up their babies for adoption through the processes of "relinquishing." As a mother who herself relinquished a child she birthed in her younger years, Snyder deftly weaves her personal story into the chapter narrative. Her story provides compelling examples of doulas who help to profoundly change the birthmother's perspective from one of shame and "disenfranchised grief" to one of celebration and pride in themselves as birth-givers and in the babies that they nurture and grow. She notes that in doing so doulas also can positively affect the birthmother's readjustment to post-relinquishment life. Quoting the adage, "If you birth from a position of power, you can parent from a position of power," Snyder asks, "If a birthmother births from a position of power, with the assistance of a doula, can she then *relinquish* from a position of power?" Susanna answers in the affirmative and provides various compelling examples of exactly how doulas help relinquishing birthmothers shift their perspectives to achieve an empowered post-relinquishment identity. "What if," Snyder wonders, "we can dare to imagine a world where the provision of doulas for birthmothers is standard practice?" Now that's a world that I would like to live in! In fact, I would like to live in a world where the provision of doulas, and midwives, for every birthing woman is standard practice. I trust and hope that this excellent book will be a major step forward in achieving that dream.

In chapter five, Jon Korfmacher and Marisha Humphries address the myriad ways in which deep relationships can develop between doulas and adolescent moms. The reader can listen in as an adolescent mother, at first resistant to the notion of a stranger being around during her labour, but after extended contact with her doula ends up saying, "Now she's, like, the only person I *want* to be there." I was especially intrigued to learn that the doula-young mother relationship often extends into postpartum care, richening and deepening after the birth because now the two share not only the birth experience in all its intimacy, but also a fascination with the baby. The doulas' art here, the authors found, is to carefully balance their attraction to holding and talking about the newborn with the mom's need for her doula to keep her attention on her, the newborn mother, as well. In their study, contact between mother and doula increased as the pregnancy progressed, peaked during labour and birth, and tapered off slowly (yet was still critical for the young moms) during the postpartum period. Doula flexibility was key throughout—the doulas needed to be flexible about when and where they met with the moms and to avoid being "too prescriptive"—for example, to be accepting should the mother choose to bottle-feed even though the doula model of care strongly promotes breastfeeding.

Amy Gilliland's chapter six describes doulas as facilitators of transformation and grief. From her chapter, I learned that pregnancy and birth-related grief can take many forms: new mothers may grieve for their lost former life, for the birth that they wanted but didn't achieve, for the baby who died or was born ill or deformed, or for a loved one who died during the pregnancy. Gilliland's interviewees experienced all these types of grief, and all of them trusted their doulas to guide them through, "to show them the way to their new life and to integrate their experiences." Doulas helped these women by acknowledging their fears and being present to their pain. As "trusted guides and wise witnesses," the doulas assisted the mothers through all of the five well-known stages of grief—here Gilliland astutely notes that these stages do not necessarily constitute a linear progression but rather are experienced more like a pendulum moving back and forth. The doulas neither blamed nor judged; they "understood the emotions of grief and did not shy away from their intensity." They encouraged the mothers to express their grief either in conversation or through journaling. They helped women to find the information that they needed—"why did my baby die?" They offered counselling, emotional support, and coping measures. They helped the mothers to bathe and dress their dead babies, and make funeral arrangements—these are all doula services of which I had previously been unaware. They offered support to family members as well. In one particularly moving story, a doula describes how she assisted a mother whose husband had died in one of the Twin Towers on 9/11 through a Caesarean birth, achieving a small miracle when she convinced the hospital staff to put the baby skin-to-skin with the mother right after the birth. To the amazement of the mother and the staff, the baby did the "breast crawl," which the doula captured on film, and when the mother looked into her baby's eyes, she saw the eyes of her husband looking up at her—a profound moment of mixed grief and joy, death, and life.

Section two of this volume focuses on doulas in community context—another topic new to me. Chapter seven's author Maria Abegunde describes herself as an ancestral priest, ritual specialist, and devotee of the Yoruba *orisa* Osun, whose task is "to care for the ancestors, those yet to be born, and the living." She writes that choosing the doula path for her has meant choosing "Yemanja, Mother of the Ocean, Protector of Women, Children.... She Who Feeds Us from the Infinite Bounty of the Sea ... like the Virgin, Yemanja turns no one away and welcomes everyone under her skirts." Abegunde carries lessons learned from Yemanja from the beach to the birthing room, where she strives to be mindful that she has entered an external womb that contains the inner womb of the mother preparing to give birth. "I have entered, therefore, a level of the cosmos and consciousness that exists between dimensions. Before I enter the room, I ready (and steady) myself by agreeing to be present but invisible: this moment—no matter how long—is not my moment."

In this lovely, mystical way, Abegunde describes how she sees and experiences the role of the doula. Listening and paying attention are her keys; synchronizing her breathing with the mother's and noting changes in the labouring woman's breathing patterns are some of her most-prized techniques. Looking into the mother's eyes, bearing witness, and offering touch are part of what she calls her "matricentric" approach to birth—I love that term! The womb and the ocean—the womb of us all, the matrix from which we all emerged—these are the tropes and the tone of her beautiful chapter. Birth, like death, is a doorway through which Yemanja's waters flow. During labour, one of the final powerful things Abegunde feels she can do as a doula is "to make certain that the mother knows before labour, during labour, and postpartum that her entire being is part of a community that holds her bodies in sacred time and space." I wish for all doulas the strong sense of the magical and mysterious that Abegunde holds so dear, that keeps her vision so clear, and that connects her to the wonders of Yemanja and of life, both before and after death.

Nicole Gallicchio begins chapter eight with the question, "What kind of doula are you?" and goes on to address the "multiple moralities" and politics of what she terms "ethical becoming." Her chapter primarily addresses (1) the fascinating risk facing doulas of overpowering rather than empowering their clients, just as the biomedical system does; and (2) the challenge to find the balance between ideology and practice that doulas must confront. Much in this chapter was new news to me. For instance, Gallicchio found during her research that the doula community she worked with defined a "good doula" not as one skilled in the use of multiple techniques or with excellent statistics, but as a doula who has something more subtle and intangible—a kind of mastery over herself, a self-awareness within and through the work. Even doulas considered "dangerous" by their community because of their political activism were still considered to be good doulas if they developed what Gallicchio aptly and innovatively calls an "expertise of the self."

I was surprised to learn that in the Pacific Coast doula community Gallicchio studied, experienced doulas regularly encouraged newcomers to reflect on the roots of any intense emotions that they felt while supporting a labouring woman, so that they could leave their own "birth baggage" at the door. I learned that there are "saviour doulas" who want to save their clients from the traumas that they experienced during birth, activist doulas who resent authority, doulas who use birth as a form of self-therapy, and doulas who want to take care of everyone because they need to be needed. There are doulas who are too attached to the romance and drama of birth to be able to be fully present for the woman, and others who are too ideologically rigid—doulas are expected in this community (and others no doubt) to embrace a flexible and fluid sense of self. So "dealing with your birth baggage" means reflecting on and then enacting self-knowledge and self-awareness to develop expertise of self. Tools for this process include rebirthing, "doula-specific psychotherapy," retreats, sweat lodges, sharing circles, and experiential body learning via vaginal exams or mapping one's pelvic region. Gallicchio notes:

> Developing this "expertise of the self" around—rather than through—the work of the doula allowed doulas to figure out for themselves how to navigate that ambiguous and amorphous line between being agential and pushing an agenda, between empowering and overpowering, and to learn how to support without supplanting.

I love that sentence! And I love the profound insightfulness of this chapter. It takes us deep into doula values, psychology, and ideology, showing us how doulas struggle to balance that ideology with hospital realities and women's own, often differing, beliefs and desires—the expertise of self that doulas work to develop in their process of "ethical becoming."

In chapter nine, Angela Castañeda and Julie Johnson Searcy address doula work as "a complex and multidimensional form of intimate labour." For them, the term *intimate labour* constitutes a useful analytical category for understanding the doula role because that intimate labour offers opportunities for embodied resistance to the homogenizing medical approach to birth. Via their physical, psychological, and emotional closeness to the labouring woman, doulas gain intimate knowledge of her and of her body. This is the first chapter in the book to address the grueling aspects of doula labour care — how physically challenging it is to provide the continuous support that produces the doula effect. I am glad to see that issue addressed as I have often wondered at the stamina doulas exhibit, providing intimate care often day after day. They use their bodies, far more than their artifacts (rebozos, ropes, etc.), to give that care, and by the end of the birth, they may have bruises, strained muscles, and total exhaustion to show for it. (I think that if I were a doula, I would have to go running to my chiropractor after every birth!) The detrimental physical effects are often compensated for by the endorphin rush that they experience when the birth goes well—they share, I think, in that emotional, and often also spiritual, high felt by all present when

---

the hormones are flowing and the presence of God or some strong spiritual force seems immanent in the room.

Boundaries are most certainly an issue as the authors show. The doula must "walk a tightrope" between offering too much intimacy and offering too little: they must develop that expertise of the self that is discussed so clearly in the preceding chapter. One of the doulas whom Castañeda and Searcy interviewed notes that she strives not to talk too much about herself because the birth and her care are not about her. She needs to be "a projection screen" so that the mother won't waste energy trying to please her. She must "hold the space" for the mother to be and do as she needs and wants.

Aptly, the authors note the tensions between the deep intimacy doulas seek to establish with their clients and the demands of the market and their profession—another tightrope doulas must walk. One doula describes this as a conflict between "the business mind and the mothering mind." Given that we live in a market economy, most doulas have to charge money for a service that women have traditionally provided for one another for free—hence the "entrepreneurial doula" who aligns with a professional organization and has to meet its bureaucratic requirements and rules. I found valuable the authors' discussion of the tensions between doulas, who see birth as a natural process and strive to keep it that way (if that's what the mother wants) and nurses, who tend to see birth as a problem waiting to happen. Some nurses note that they wish to, but cannot, provide doula care because of the many interventions that they perform and the constant charting required, which keep them from connecting with the mother as deeply as the doula can. When she subtly whispers to the husband or mother that the doctor is preparing to do the episiotomy they didn't want, the doula is practising *embodied resistance* (another useful term new to me); she is walking the tightrope between getting thrown out of the labour room and staying to provide that intimate, embodied labour experience.

Boundaries are also a major focus of chapter ten, only this time the emphasis is on postpartum doula care. Author Jacqueline Kelleher often provides doula care for as long as three months after the birth, developing intimacy with the mother's family and friends. (I can only wish that postpartum doulas had been around three decades ago when I had my children—I could really have used their help!) She finds that her voice is powerful for the family, so she strives to keep up with the latest information on infant feeding and newborn characteristics and needs. Kelleher provides *anticipatory guidance*—yet another term both new and informative for me. Over the past twenty years, she has supported hundreds of new families on their parenthood journey and notes that she has had to establish clear boundaries about her role (it does not include childcare, housecleaning, or supporting unsafe parenting practices) and with herself: not bringing her personal baggage into the family's home, not superimposing her own objectives over those of the family, and not diagnosing or treating illness. Rather, she "walks alongside" the parents, helping them to recognize when things are not normal and to find information and community resources.

Section three of this volume addresses doulas and institutions. Why do doulas matter? Vania Smith-Oka's chapter eleven provides a different sort of answer to this question by describing what labour and birth can look like in doulas' absence. She worked in an underfunded, understaffed, and overstrained Mexican public hospital where women are moved as quickly as possible through an assembly-line birthing process. While conducting ethnographic research in the hospital's maternity ward, Vania found herself becoming an "unexpected doula," offering various forms of labour support to women who otherwise had none. This hospital, located in Puebla, processes over nine thousand births per year and has a Caesarean rate of 45 percent. Pain medication is available only to Caesarean patients yet Pitocin is ubiquitous. All labouring women are forced to stay prone for their entire labour, all have IVs, and all are repeatedly examined for cervical dilation. They labour alone, are given no information, have no decision-making power, and are scolded if they do not comply with orders. Doctors often deliberately stretch their cervixes to speed the birth and pull babies out manually—both procedures cause excruciating pain. Smith-Oka (who had taken a doula training course between fieldwork stints) did her best to alleviate their terror and pain; she held hands, gazed into women's eyes, and rubbed their backs. Most importantly, Smith-Okia argues for the inclusion of doulas in the Mexican public health care system.

I cannot help but contrast this Mexican public hospital with a public hospital in Belo Horizonte, Minas Gerais, Brazil, called Hospital Sofia Feldman. There, doulas are fully incorporated into the system; the hospital provides them at no charge to any birthing mother who arrives unaccompanied. When family members do come, a few are welcome to stay, even though there is very little space for them in the tiny cubicles women occupy during labour. IVs are not mandatory, Pitocin is rarely used, and women walk the halls and the lovely small gardens freely during labour. That hospital too is poor in resources yet manages nevertheless to provide thoroughly humanized care (Georges and Davis-Floyd, "Humanistic Obstetrics in Brazil"). As I have so often argued, it's ideology, not resources, that determines how women are treated during labour and birth. There can be no better example of why doulas matter than showing what the *lack* of doulas means for women in this, and so many other, public hospitals in the global South.

In contrast to the tension between nurses and doulas described in chapter nine, the four authors of chapter twelve examine possibilities for *collaboration* between the two groups—a welcome contrast. The authors—Christine Morton, Marla Seacrist, Jennifer Torres, and Nicole Heidbreder—found that most of the nurses in their study agreed that doulas did enhance the labour experience for the mother, and many felt that doulas are collaborative team members. The authors interpret these findings as "cautious support" for doulas among nurses, but only when doulas stay within their labour support role. Many nurses truly appreciated the presence of the doula, as they knew that the woman would continue to have support when they had to leave her room; they were also supportive of the doulas who advocated for the staff to follow the mother's written birth plan. The doulas surveyed tended to feel positive about nurses and to see them as collaborative and not interfering with the doula-client relationship. The doulas reported trying hard to be helpful to the nurses by assisting the mother to the bathroom, for example, and working equally hard to avoid being tagged as a "bad doula" who resists procedures or provides contradictory information. Interestingly, newbie nurses were often intimidated by experienced doulas and vice-versa.

Strategies conducive to greater collaboration between nurses and doulas suggested by the authors and their interviewees included the following: having doulas shadow a nurse as part of their training; educating nurses about the role of the doula; allowing more information sharing between nurses and doulas; giving mutual assessment of each other's level of experience; and having patience with both newbie doulas and newbie nurses. For nurses accustomed to epidural labours, doulas can model how to care for a woman having a natural birth, and nurses can be trained in labour support techniques so that they can use them themselves and can understand what doulas are doing when they use such techniques. Wondering why nurses' views of doulas were less positive than doula's views of nurses, the authors looked for explanatory factors and found that nurses who most enjoy providing labour support tended to have the most positive view of doulas. That might be, I presume, because they value and appreciate labour support in general.

In chapter thirteen, authors Annie Robinson and Lauren Mitchell focus on "Story-Centred Care: Full-Spectrum Doula Work and Narrative Medicine." They begin with a compelling narrative about Robinson's attendance at an abortion and proceed to describe the *full-spectrum doula movement*; it consists of doulas that "provide care at no cost to individuals across the spectrum of pregnancy choices, including during abortions, miscarriages, stillbirth inductions, adoption planning, and births for low-income women." Part of "The Doula Project," these full-spectrum doulas partner with institutions to stand as advocates and supporters of women. They believe that disconnection between patients and caregivers can be repaired via promoting the art of storytelling during clinical interactions—another surprise for me! They note, "We consider the principles and practice of narrative medicine to be the foundation on and materials out of which full-spectrum doula support is built."

As a folklorist, I know that stories give meaning and coherence to experience, so I can understand the importance of telling and listening to stories in health care. Facts are objective; stories are deeply personal. Simply listening to people's stories can validate their interpretations of their experience; narrating the story can help to generate those interpretations. Because doulas are non-medical caregivers, they have more time than medical personnel to listen to stories and to have conversations that aid in infusing the stories and the experiences they recount with coherent meaning. Felicitously, the authors address *caregivers'* needs to tell stories as well. In a deeply compassionate and intuitive paragraph, the authors say:

> We have often witnessed providers walk into a day of procedures still feeling wounded by the questions or doubts in clinical judgment from the previous patient. Caregivers take their patients' decisions—and their pain—very personally. And thus, to protect oneself and one's capacity to continue working, providers often begin to seek objectivity so much that the pain dissolves.

The authors stress that doulas working as part of institutions can provide support to that young resident grappling with the emotions of performing an abortion, or even, I would add, to that seasoned OB who has just lost a mother to a sudden hemorrhage or amniotic fluid embolism. The process of writing or speaking one's story can be healing for caregivers suffering from compassion fatigue as well as for patients suffering from illness and pain. Comical stories provide needed release in laughter; tragic stories can enable the teller to let go of the pain. And what the authors term *narrative humility* can enable us to listen to others' stories and accept that we cannot ever fully share their experience or even fully understand it, but we *can* be present, open, and accepting of their need to speak and be heard.

Chapter fourteen, by Courtney Everson and Melissa Cheyney, opens our eyes to the concepts of *liminality* (the threshold state of being "betwixt and between") and *mandorla spaces* (Johnson and Davis-Floyd "Home to Hospital Transport"). A *mandorla* is that magical space at the intersection of two circles (or paradigms, or ideologies) in which opposites can meet and harmoniously interact. The authors argue that because of their liminality—the fact that they stand on a threshold between the medical and midwifery models of care—doulas can create and inhabit this mandorla space in harmonious interaction with medical personnel.

Five themes emerged from their analysis of doula care models as described by various birth-related organizations: (1) doulas as specialists in the psychosocial needs of childbearing women; (2) support of physiologic birth; (3) provision of individualized, evidence-based support; (4) facilitation of communication and relationship; (5) continuous companionship. These key themes are essential elements of the doula model of care. They also reveal the liminal nature of the mandorla space created between the medical and midwifery paradigms. The authors see doulas as mediators between these two paradigms, holding open a space where the power of the in-between may be co-opted and used to instigate social transformation. *Doulas as agitators* can disrupt the routine flow of technocratic births, creating tensions between the doula and the hospital staff; *doulas as facilitators* of hospital birth can create tensions with homebirth midwives, who see the doula as enabling women to accept technocratic births by softening and humanizing them, thereby allowing the "oppression" to endure.

The authors argue that in occupying that liminal space between the medical and midwifery (or technocratic and holistic) paradigms, doulas can bring elements of each into the other and serve as a bridge between these two worlds. As labouring women receive compassion and support from their doulas, they "may begin a process of unlearning and relearning, emerging confident in the power of their own bodies, of physiologic birth, and of the role women caring for women can play in Caesarean reduction and healthy outcomes for mother and baby." This relearning may have a powerful effect on subsequent birth choices by opening a wider path to midwife-led home and birth-centre births and by generating a subtle yet transformative revolution in women's birth choices from within the heart of the doula mandorla.

In chapter fifteen, "Reimagining the Birthing Body: Reproductive Justice and New Directions in Doula Care," Monica Basile affirms this suggestion when she notes that doulas see themselves as effecting change "one birth at a time." More broadly, Basile seeks to understand how the doula movement contributes to human rights and social justice through challenging inequalities of race, class, gender, and sexuality. One doula she interviewed stated "when women reclaim the right to birth on their own terms, they might feel more empowered to challenge other forms of discrimination and repression." She introduces the *reproductive justice doula*, who seeks to address maternity care disparities tied to racism and socio-economic marginalization—e.g., the higher rates of premature births and mortality for African-American babies in the U.S. Her reproductive justice doulas consist of community-based doulas, prison doulas, full-spectrum doulas, and radical doulas. She argues that these new directions in doula care are generating productive and vital links between reproductive health care and social justice advocacy.

Community-based doulas tend to be of the same racial or ethnic background as their clients and work to support the women—often the young, poor, and underprivileged— of their communities. They see supporting individual women as akin to supporting the entire neighborhood. *Prison doulas* provide classes to prisoners, care during birth, postpartum support that focuses on helping women cope with separation from their babies, and community networking around the prisoners' issues and needs. Basile also adds a focus on full-spectrum doulas and their work in supporting women through pregnancy loss.

When I first saw the term *radical doula* in this chapter, I imagined that it might mean something similar to the term *renegade midwife*—a midwife who places the desires of the woman ahead of the interests of the profession, often attending births that are out of protocol and would generally be considered too dangerous to take place at home (Davis-Floyd "Renegade Midwives"). I was wrong! A radical doula turns out to be one who embraces multiplicity of identity and is committed to making doula care available to marginalized women, such as immigrants, LGBTQ people, teen mothers, drug users, abuse survivors, and single and low-income parents. These doulas argue for humanized treatment of individual women and of marginalized populations within a reproductive justice ideology. Some of these doulas are male, trans, gender nonconforming, and genderqueer. They recognize the importance of shared identities between doula and client. They advocate for greater racial diversity within the doula community and greater understanding of issues of racism and privilege as they relate to birthing politics and practices. Many come through the International Center for Traditional Childbearing's (ICTC) Full Circle doula training program. They bear witness to "overlapping forms of social injustice and birth injustice" and seek to combine birthwork with social justice activism. They are changing the narrow, binary (medical-midwifery) frame within which the effects of medicalization are understood by shifting to a broader focus on equality, access, and justice.

Want to know what doulas do? Why they matter? Where they fit inside our communities and within our larger U.S. health care system? What challenges they face? What triumphs they have achieved? And what their future might look like? Read this gem of a book!

WORKS CITED

Davis-Floyd, Robbie. "The Technocratic, Humanistic, and Holistic Models of Birth." *International Journal of Gynecology & Obstetrics* 75., Supplement No. 1 (2001): S5-S23. Print.

Davis-Floyd, Robbie. *Birth as an American Rite of Passage.* Berkeley: University of California Press, 2004 [1992]. Print.

Davis-Floyd, Robbie. "Renegade Midwives: Assets or Liabilities?" *Mainstreaming Midwives: The Politics of Change.* Eds. Robbie Davis-Floyd and Christine Barbara Johnson. New York: Routledge, 2006. 447-468. Print.

Davis-Floyd, Robbie and Eugenia Georges. "Humanistic Obstetrics in Brazil: A Revolution in Maternity Care." *The Routledge Handboook of Medical Anthropology.* Eds. Lenore Manderson, Anita Hardon, and Elizabeth Cartwright. London: Routledge, 2016. Print.

Davis-Floyd, Robbie and Charles Laughlin. *The Power of Ritual.* Brisbane, Australia: Daily Grail Publishing, 2016. Print.

Johnson, Christine Barbara and Robbie Davis-Floyd. "Home to Hospital Transport: Fractured Articulations or Magical Man-

dorlas?" *Mainstreaming Midwives: The Politics of Change*. Eds.
Robbie Davis-Floyd and Christine Barbara Johnson. New York:
Routledge, 2006. 469-506. Print.

Introduction

Across the Reproductive Divide

ANGELA N. CASTAÑEDA AND JULIE JOHNSON SEARCY

FTER THE BIRTH OF OUR FIRST CHILDREN in 2008, we separately found ourselves on the path to become doulas. The intense and transformative nature of birth captivated us and seemed an arena to nourish the interest that we both already had in women's issues. We found supporting women in their transition to motherhood widely appealing, especially as we negotiated our own transition as parents. Shortly after formal training, we started advertising our services as doulas and taking on clients. Our services included going into women's homes before their labour began, discussing their birth options with them, and then returning to provide physical and emotional comfort when they began to labour. Most women we worked with gave birth in the hospital, and as doulas we accompanied them in their transition from home to hospital. We each had our own separate experiences as we began attending births in the role of doula, but we began talking and reflecting on what it was like to be a doula from both personal and anthropological perspectives. We supported each other as we experienced the stress of being on-call and never knowing when a mom might go into labour, as we encountered uncertainty in our role as doula in a hospital setting, and as we shared different comfort measures that seemed to help women. We also observed and discussed the dynamics between doulas within our community and talked about what was required to professionalize as a doula.

As academics, we looked to social science scholarship for some critical distance and insight about the work that we were doing as doulas. Had anyone written about the embodied work of being a doula? What had social scientists discovered about the tensions and boundaries in the various relationships doulas navigate? We found important contributions in dissertation research on doulas from Christine Morton (*Doula Care*) and Cheryl Hunter (*The Doula as Educator*), but this research only left us searching for more. We found a number of studies that considered the medical efficacy of doulas (Scott et al.; Zhang et al.; Campbell et al.; Campbell et al.), and of course we read the work on doulas by Drs. John H. Kennell and Marshall H. Klaus ("Continuous Emotions Support;" *Mothering the Mother*; "The Doula;" *The Doula Book*), but we were still hoping for more dialogue from the social sciences on the role of doulas in reproduction (Norman and Rothman). It was this opening in academic scholarship and our own richly textured experience as doulas that led us to begin research on doulas in our community, which eventually led to this book.

Now the cultural landscape is changing, and we hear much more about doulas in academic circles and in popular culture. Today, doulas routinely emerge in mainstream media (*NYT*, *WSJ*) and often appear in or are referenced on TV shows (*About a Boy*, *Jane the Virgin*, *Mulaney*, and *Bones*). In 2011, National Public Radio ran a four-month series called the "Baby Project." The stories followed nine women across the United States as they made decisions about birthing their children. The stories covered the discussions and debates surrounding reproductive technologies, birth location, pain relief, method of birth, birth attendants including doulas, and parenting practices. The "Baby Project" was unusual in the way it sought to cover a spectrum of experiences around pregnancy, birth and parenting, and in the way it brought these experiences to mainstream media. Other major news agencies such as *The New York Times* have also covered a number of stories about doulas and the work they do with birthing women (Wilgoren; Paul; Rochman; Hartocollis). Reproductive issues are important topics in the media for their ability to reveal how societies imagine what it means to be a person, how people come into being, and ultimately what it means for a society to reproduce itself (Ginsburg and Rapp; Kauffman and Morgan; Franklin). Too often the cultural tone around discussions on reproduction centre on binaries—home or hospital, cesarean or vaginal, non-medicated or medicated. In highlighting the role of the doula, this book helps to move away from these binaries and helps to regain a sense of fluidity around birth. Thinking about birth through the lens of the doula allows us to raise questions about the nature of birth and the social actors involved in the culturally critical moments of reproduction. This book looks at the embodied and intimate labour doulas perform at birth.

Klaus, Kennell, and Klaus define a doula as a "woman experienced in childbirth who provides continuous physical, emotional and information support to the mother before, during and just after childbirth" (3). Today doulas work to support women across a reproductive spectrum. They provide their services to women experiencing abortions, adoption, incarceration, stillbirth, miscarriages, and to women during the postpartum period. Doulas provide emotional, physical, informational advocacy, and they help in negotiating relationships between family, friends, and care providers (Gilliland). Doulas have no clinical training and are non-medical professionals, but a growing body of research suggests that the presence of a doula supports physiological birth and healthier outcomes for mothers and babies (Hodnett; Hodnett et al.). As Megan Davidson, a doula and contributor in this volume suggests, doulas "seek to reduce fear and build confidence, increase knowledge and informed decision making, offer practical support and advocacy to women." The very nature of doulas' intimate labour provides a unique analytic to engage the often-contentious debates around reproductive care. Doulas move in and out of private and public places and build relationships that traverse families and institutions. Our goal in crafting this volume is to highlight the ways in which doulas operate in liminal spaces and engage in intimate labour. Doulas also provide a unique way to think through the complexities surrounding reproduction because of the embodied intimate nature of the labour that they provide and their ability to navigate between and across boundaries.

DOULAS: PAST AND PRESENT

Prior to the medicalization of birth in industrialized countries, women supported one another during their childbirth and postpartum period (Raphael; Leavitt). Doulas in their current form emerged from the 1970s women's health movement. As midwives watched the professionalization of medicine in North America, obstetricians and hospitals became the standard of care for women giving birth, and the practice of women supporting one another during childbirth disappeared (Leavitt). The women's health movement in the 1970s drew critical attention to highly medicalized births and clinical practices around reproduction (Phillips; Morgen). Scholars such as Barbara Katz Rothman and Robbie Davis-Floyd drew on the work of the women's health movement to outline a midwifery model of care and a technocratic or medicalized model of care for birthing women that were most often at odds with each other. These critiques of health reproduction offered up "natural" childbirth and homebirth as alternatives to the routinized, medicalized, and high-intervention births. The practices of homebirth, midwifery, and childbirth education classes and a return to women-supported labour emerged out of, and in response to, the women's health movement.

From the Greek word *doule*, meaning female slave, helper, or maidservant (Merriam-Webster), the term doula entered academic literature in 1973 when medical anthropologist Dana Raphael used the word in her book *The Tender Gift* to describe the importance of supporting a new mother for successful breastfeeding results. During this same period, Drs. John Kennell and Marshall Klaus conducted clinical trials on maternal-infant bonding and determined that the continual support of a doula not only benefitted bonding but also decreased complications. Together with Penny Simkin, Phyllis Klaus, and Annie Kennedy, Drs. Kennell and Klaus founded in 1992 the first professional doula organization, Doulas of North America DONA International. As women recognized the positive impact continuous emotional and physical support could bring to women in labour, more women came to work as doulas, and professional organizations began to create training and certification programs. An Internet search reveals over twenty professional organizations now exist to train, certify, and support doulas. Each of these organizations has its own take on what is required to train and certify a doula, but all these programs acknowledge the embodied and relational labour at the heart of doula work.

RELATIONAL AND INTIMATE LABOUR

Sociologist Barbara Katz Rothman asked, "What would it mean to live in a culture that values relationships?" in her keynote address "Women as Fathers" for the New Maternalisms: Tales of Motherwork conference held in New York City in April of 2015. Her question underscores Western culture's tendency to devalue social relationships, and it highlights the need for further analysis on labour rooted in relationships, such as doula work,. The chapters in this volume emphasize the relational and intimate labour of doulas. Doulas engage in what Viviana Zelizer defines as "relational work," connecting the economic transactions with their crafting of social relationships (35). At the same time, doulas also work in intensely intimate spaces.

Intimate labour is a useful lens to understand the tension in doula work that is described as both internal and material. Eileen Boris and Rhacel Salazar Parreñas define intimate labour as "work that involves embodied and affective interactions in the service of social reproduction" (7). It involves bridging intimate care from both within and outside of an individual's home. Doulas negotiate boundaries and often blur the divisions between communities and across public and private spheres in their practice of intimate labour. This book weaves together three main threads: doulas and mothers, doulas and their community, and finally, doulas and institutions. The lived experience of doulas illustrates the interlacing relationships between all three of these threads.

The essays in this collection offer a unique perspective on doulas by bringing together voices that represent the full spectrum of doula work, including the viewpoints of birth, postpartum, abortion, community based, adoption, prison, and radical doulas. We privilege this broad representation of doula experiences to emphasize the importance of a multi-vocal framing of the doula experience. Although the papers in this volume represent the spectrum of doula roles, we acknowledge the dominant North American context. It is our hope that this volume invites dialogue on the spectrum of doula labour from a more global perspective.

This volume also values the diversity of voices and includes personal reflections from doulas on their everyday experiences with intimate labour as well as academic analysis of doula work. From the theoretical insights of junior and senior scholars in anthropology, Black studies, psychology, social work, sociology, and women's studies to the experiences of practising doulas, midwives, and nurses, the essays in this collection serve to bridge the gap between lived and theoretical understandings of doula experiences. The diversity of disciplines represented in these chapters also lends itself to the use of multiple descriptors for the work doulas do. Although authors use both care and labour to describe this work, all of the chapters draw attention to the relationship between doulas and intimacy within reproduction.

In section one, "Doulas and Mothers," six chapters highlight the intricate relationship between doulas and the women that they serve.[1] This section begins by reviewing the scholarly evidence for doula-supported births. A practising doula in New York City and a cultural anthropologist, Megan Davidson's essay pairs the lived and the theoretical in chapter one. She reviews the literature that demonstrates positive outcomes for mothers and babies when doulas are present, and she adds important ethnographic evidence to this scholarship. In chapter two, "Retrieving the Maps to Motherhood," Alison Bastien draws on her thirty years of experience as a midwife, doula, and childbirth educator to challenge the role that doulas play as they work with women in labour. In chapter three, Sarah Lewin, a clinical social worker and doula, provides another cautionary example of the doula-mother relationship. Lewin dissects the impact of contemporary U.S. body culture on pregnant women and on the doulas who serve them. In chapter four, Susanna Snyder's exploratory piece raises questions about the way doulas may help birth mothers cope with grief when relinquishing a baby, and she addresses the doula's ability to counter powerful cultural narratives that cast these mothers as deviant. Community-based doulas are the focus in chapter five by Jon Korfmacher and Marisha Humphries, whose work looks at how the relationship between doulas and teenage mothers changes over time. In the final chapter of this section, chapter six, Amy Gilliland examines the role that doulas play in transforming the grief mothers experience around birth.

Section two, "Doulas and Their Community" extends the scope

of relational labour to include essays that examine the kinds of complex relationships doulas have with one another as well as reflexive accounts of their own work. This section highlights an inward focused approach to doula work, as illustrated in "Learning to Walk in Water: Invoking Yemanja on the Doula Path." In this chapter, Abegunde documents her spiritual journey through doula work framed by her experience as an *egungun* (ancestral) priest. The reflexive nature of the doula experience is further analyzed in chapter eight by Nicole Gallicchio, which focuses on the importance of an "expertise of self" as a required characteristic of doulas. In our chapter, chapter nine, we investigate the multiple ways bodies are materialized through the intimate practices of doulaing and birthing. We address how doulas simultaneously use the fluidity of their own bodies to cross borders from intimate to institutional settings while we also highlight the importance of a personalized birthing body. In chapter ten, the final chapter for this section, postpartum doula Jacqueline Kelleher emphasizes the importance of defining and maintaining boundaries with new families via the specialized work involved in postpartum care.

In section three, "Doulas and Institutions," we broaden the spectrum of doula care to include the intricate relationships that doulas negotiate within institutional spaces. In chapter eleven, Vania Smith-Oka's research in Mexico pushes the boundaries of doula work by analyzing the experience of birthing in spaces where women have little control over their birth experiences. Her chapter addresses provider-patient interactions, including between midwives and obstetricians, and she identifies "microsupport" as a way for doulas to allow labouring women "to feel cared for and supported in a chaotic birth environment." In chapter twelve, written by Christine Morton, Marla Seacrist, Jennifer Torres and Nicole Heidbreder, the relationship between doulas and labour and delivery nurses is examined by focusing on how doulas carefully navigate and negotiate boundaries. Annie Robinson and Lauren Mitchell use narrative medicine in "Story-Centered Care" to document their experiences as full-spectrum doulas. Their work flows across the spectrum of pregnancy choices, including abortions, miscarriages, stillbirth inductions, adoption planning, and births for low-income individuals. In chapter fourteen, Courtney Everson and Melissa

Cheyney's essay identifies doula care as operating in a *mandorla* space between hospital-based obstetrics and homebirth midwifery. In this liminal position, doulas serve as "transitional birthing professionals" to help bridge different birth communities. And in the last chapter, "Reimagining the Birthing Body," Monica Basile encourages us to move beyond the doula-institution relationship to reconsider the other ways doulas engage with larger issues of reproductive justice. Basile argues that, "doulas are increasingly working from a political consciousness that perceives birthing choices as part of the spectrum of reproductive rights, and as tied to struggles for social justice and human rights."

CONCLUSION

Scholars turn to reproduction for its ability to illuminate the practices involved with negotiating personhood for the unborn, the newborn, and the already-existing family members, community members, and the nation. The scholarship in this volume draws attention to doula work as intimate and relational while highlighting the way boundaries are created, maintained, challenged, and transformed. Intimate labour as a theoretical construct provides a way to think about the kind of care doulas offer women across the reproductive spectrum. As doulas attend to women's physical and emotional needs, they develop relationships that Zelizer defines as intimate:

> We can think of relations as intimate to the extent that interactions within them depend on particularized knowledge received, and attention provided by, at least one person. The knowledge involved includes such elements as shared secrets, interpersonal rituals, bodily information, and awareness of personal vulnerability. (3)

As the work in this volume demonstrates, doulas gain intimate knowledge about the women whom they work with as they see them through the physically vulnerable act of birth, abortion, adoption, and their aftermath. Paying attention to the kind of work doulas perform opens up a scholarly space to consider how intimate labour materializes bodies and guides people through transitions. Working doulas in this volume call attention to the way intimate labour requires a mindfulness of self and other; scholars in this volume point out the way intimate labour requires doulas to straddle a space between the intimate and the public—like mothers, they move between boundaries, inside and outside of different spaces, and across thresholds.

This volume comes just as scholarly interest in doulas is beginning to swell—at a moment when the cultural impact of doulas is apparent from media and news agencies. As doulas move between worlds and learn to live in liminal spaces, they occupy space that allows them to generate new cultural narratives about birthing bodies. Critical analysis of doulas as they both encounter and redefine boundaries suggests new ways of approaching maternity care and reproduction reform. It also demonstrates larger social debates at stake in the discussions surrounding maternal care. We hope that this volume will serve as the impetus for further discussion about doulas and what a powerful analytic they can be in expanding the debates on reproduction.

ENDNOTE

[1]For more detailed description of chapters, please see foreword.

WORKS CITED

Boris, Eileen and Rhacel Salazar Parreñas. "Introduction." *Intimate Labors: Cultures,Technologies, and the Politics of Care.* Eds. Eileen Boris and Rhacel Salazar Parreñas. Stanford, CA: Stanford University Press, 2010. 1-17. Print.

Campbell, Della A. et al. "A Randomized Control Trial of Continuous Support in Labor by a Lay Doula." *Journal of Obstetric, Gynecologic, & Neonatal Nursing* 35.4 (2006): 456-464. Print.

Campbell, Della A. et al. "Female Relatives or Friends Trained as Labor Doulas: Outcomes at 6 to 8 Weeks Postpartum." *Birth* 34.3 (2007): 220-227. Print.

Davis-Floyd, Robbie. *Birth as An American Rite of Passage.* Berkeley: University of California Press, 1992. Print.

"Doula." *Merriam-Webster*. Merriam-Webster, 2015. Web. 25 May 2015.

Franklin, Sarah. *Embodied Progress: A Cultural Account of Assisted Conception*. New York: Routledge, 2002. Print.

Gilliland, Amy. "After Praise and Encouragement: Emotional Support Strategies Used by Birth Doulas in the USA and Canada." *Midwifery* 27.4 (2011): 525-531. Print.

Ginsburg, Faye D., and Rayna Rapp, eds. *Conceiving the New World Order: The Global Politics of Reproduction*. Berkeley: University of California Press, 1995. Print.

Hartocollis, Anemona. "Doulas, A Growing Force in Maternity Culture, Seek Greater Acceptance." *New York Times* 11 February 2015: A20. Print.

Hodnett ED. "Pain and Women's Satisfaction with the Experience of Childbirth: A Systematic Review." *American Journal of Obstetrics and Gynecology* 186.5 (2002): S160-S172. Print.

Hodnett, ED et al. "Continuous Support for Women during Childbirth (Review)." *The Cochrane Database of Systematic Reviews* 2 (2011). Print.

Hunter, Cheryl. *The Doula as Educator: Labor, Embodiment and Intimacy in Childbirth*. Diss. Indiana University, 2007. Ann Arbor: ProQuest/UMI, 2007. Print.

Kaufman, Sharon R. and Lynn M. Morgan. "The Anthropology of the Beginnings and Ends of life." *Annual Review of Anthropology* 34 (2005): 317-341. Print.

Kennell, John et al. "Continuous Emotional Support during Labor in a U.S. Hospital: A Randomized Controlled Trial." *Jama* 265.17 (1991): 2197-2201. Print.

Klaus, Marshall H., John H. Kennell and Phyllis H. Klaus. *Mothering the Mother: How a Doula Can Help You Have a Shorter, Easier and Healthier Birth*. Cambridge, MA: Perseus Books, 1993. Print.

Klaus, M. H., and J. H. Kennell. "The Doula: an Essential Ingredient of Childbirth Rediscovered." *Acta Paediatrica* 86.10 (1997): 1034-1036. Print.

Klaus, M. H., and J. H. Kennell. *The Doula Book: How a Trained Labor Companion Can Help You Have a Shorter, Easier, and Healthier Birth*. Cambridge, MA: Perseus Books, 2002. Print.

Leavitt, Judith Walzer. *Brought to Bed: Childbearing in America, 1750 to 1950*. New York: Oxford University Press, 1986. Print.

Morgen, Sandra. *Into Our Own Hands: The Women's Health Movement in the United States, 1969-1990*. New Brunswick, NJ: Rutgers University Press, 2002. Print.

Morton, Christine. *Doula Care: The (Re)-Emergence of Woman-Supported Childbirth in the United States*. Diss. UCLA, 2002. Ann Arbor: ProQuest/UMI, 2002. Print.

Norman, Bari Meltzer and Barbara Katz Rothman. "The New Arrival: Labor Doulas and the Fragmentation of Midwifery and Caregiving." *Laboring on: Birth in transition in the United States*. Eds. Wendy Simonds, Barbara Katz Rothman, and Bari Meltzer Norman. New York: Taylor & Francis, 2007. 251-282. Print.

Paul, Pamela. "And the Doula Makes Four." *New York Times* 2 March 2008. Fashion and Style. Print.

Phillips, Jill. *Our Bodies, Ourselves a Health Book by and for Women*. New York: Simon and Schuster, 1973. Print.

Raphael, Dana. *The Tender Gift: Breastfeeding*. Englewood Cliffs, NJ: Prentice-Hall, 1973. Print.

Rochman, Bonnie. "Men at Work for Women in Labor." *New York Times* 3 December 2013: D6. Print.

Rothman, Barbara Katz. *In Labor: Women and Power in the Birthplace*. New York Norton, 1982. Print.

Scott, Kathryn D., Gale Berkowitz, and Marshall Klaus. "A Comparison of Intermittent and Continuous Support During Labor: A Meta-Analysis." *American Journal of Obstetrics and Gynecology* 180.5 (1999): 1054-1059. Print.

Simkin, Penny. "The Birth Doula's Contribution to Modern Maternity Care." Dona International Position Paper. 2012. Print.

Wilgoren, Jodi. "'Mothering the Mother' During Childbirth, and After." *New York Times* 25 September 2005. Print.

Zhang, Jun, et al. "Continuous Labor Support from Labor Attendant for Primiparous Women: A Meta-analysis." *Obstetrics & Gynecology* 88.4 (1996): 739-744. Print.

Zelizer, Viviana. "Caring Everywhere." *Intimate Labors: Cultures, Technologies, and the Politics of Care*. Eds. Eileen Boris and Rhacel Salazar Parreñas. Stanford, CA: Stanford University Press, 2010. 267-279. Print.

I.
Doulas and Mothers

1.
Experts in Birth

How Doulas Improve Outcomes for Birthing Women and Their Babies

MEGAN DAVIDSON

"IF A DOULA WERE A DRUG, it would be unethical not to use it" (DONA 1). Birth advocates widely repeat this statement as it suggests that a medical intervention as effective as doulas would be prescribed universally. However, I argue that this points to the very model of birth that makes it difficult to accept doulas. Comparing the efficacy of doulas to drugs draws on a model of women's bodies as in need of repair or medical assistance. Martin, Gaskin, and Davis-Floyd have all aptly described this view of the female body as one where women are machines, full of shortcomings and defects, with doctors as the mechanics or technicians who fix them with science and technology, making birth both possible and safe. Davis-Floyd has written, "most routine obstetrical procedures have little or no scientific evidence to justify them" yet they continue to be "routinely performed not because they make scientific sense but because they make cultural sense" (S7). These medical interventions make sense to us culturally because they fit the model of women's bodies and of birth described above. Yet, the abundance of data showing that doulas significantly reduce the use of medical interventions sharply contrasts this cultural understanding of women's bodies and of birth.

For over two decades, medical researchers have concluded that when doulas are present the rate of vaginal births increases, labours are shorter overall, less pain medications and epidurals are requested, and vacuums or forceps are used less often. Even with all this data, only about five to six percent of births in the U.S. are attended by doulas (Morton and Clift 32; "Choices" 1), and the impact of doulas on birth and their role in the hospital with doctors and staff is rife with questions and contention (Paul 1; Gilliand 765-6). Although medical data supports the presence of a doula during labour and birth, doctors and nurses are not always as supportive (Hwang 1). Little has been written about the lived experiences of doulas or how their results are achieved in practice within the social sciences (Morton; Perez and Snedeker), and what has been written is not all positive (Norman and Rothman).

That doula support is so underutilized, resisted, and misrepresented suggests that more than clinical data is needed to help evidence the significant benefits of having doulas at all births. Although the published medical data on doulas documents numerous improvements for mothers and their infants, it does little for our knowledge of what actions account for these differences. To fill this gap, I draw from my own research with professional, experienced doulas from around the country, and I detail their specific methods, tactics, strategies, and practices. Seeking to better understand the benefits of doula support, I queried over fifty doulas throughout the U.S. I asked them specifically what they do with clients prenatally and at their births that increases the rate of vaginal deliveries, decreases the need for pain medication, and increases APGAR scores for newborns.

In what follows, I pair the mounting body of medical data showing the benefits of doula support with narratives from experienced doulas: fleshing out the impact that doula assistance has on birth outcomes for mothers and babies. First, I review the last two decades of medical data on doulas and recent endorsements by major U.S. medical associations and then I present my own research, expanding the existing literature on doula support with better ethnographic data. I detail the support that doulas cite as central to improved outcomes, such as providing prenatal education for clients, helping clients select a care provider, keeping clients calm and mobile before and during labour, and advocating for clients in a fragmented health care system. I conclude with an analysis of doulas as experts in birth who have unique practices and perspectives that help them improve birth for both mothers and babies.

MEDICAL EVIDENCE: TWO DECADES OF DATA ON DOULAS

Clinical data affirming the significant impact doulas can have on improving birth outcomes are not new. In 1993, Klaus, Kennell, and Klaus analyzed already-published data on labour support in *Mothering the Mother.* They found that doula support resulted in a 50 percent reduction in Caesarean sections, a 25 percent reduction in labour time, a 60 percent reduction in requests for epidurals, and a 40 percent reduction in pitocin use, among other impressive results (31-52). Six years later another meta-analysis (Scott, Berkowitz, Klaus) updated this data and offered new statistics: a 51 percent reduction in Caesarean sections; shorter labour time by approximately 90 minutes; a 36 percent reduction in pain medication use; and a 71 percent reduction in pitocin use (1054-9). In 2012, Klaus, Kennell, and Klaus cited new data indicating that doula support shortened labour time by 25 percent, reduced Caesarean sections by 45 percent, reduced the use of synthetic oxytocin by 40 percent; reduced the use of pain medications by 30 percent, and increased breastfeeding success and positive reports from mothers about how they felt about themselves and their infants (80; Gurevich 19-38). Similarly, in 2012, a Cochrane Review (Hodnett et al.) found that with doula support women have more spontaneous vaginal births, less pain medication, shorter labour time, fewer Cesarean sections, fewer instrumental vaginal deliveries, and their babies have higher APGAR scores. In addition to these clinically significant improvements for mothers and babies, the authors also found no reported adverse effects from having a doula, and they conclude that, "all women should have support throughout labour and birth" (6).

In 2013, Gruber, Cupito, and Dobson wrote, "the evidence suggests that it is likely more than the emotional, physical, and informational support doulas give to women during the birthing process that accounts for the reduced need for clinical procedures during labour and birth, fewer birth complications, and more satisfying experiences during labour, birth, and postpartum" (50). They state that some of the success associated with doula support is likely because doulas work as "a mother's advocate, providing a woman a sympathetic but informed ear for the choices that the birthing staff may ask her to make during the birthing process" (50). By helping clients to make informed choices, they argue, doulas allow women to make better choices that lead to improved outcomes.

Most recently, in 2014, the American College of Obstetricians & Gynecologists (ACOG) and the Society for Maternal-Fetal Medicine (SMFM) released a groundbreaking statement on preventing primary Caeserean deliveries; one of their key recommendations was doula support. They state, "Published data indicate that one of the most effective tools to improve labor and delivery outcomes is the continuous presence of support personnel, such as a doula" and conclude that, "this resource is probably underutilized" (13). Being a "probably underutilized" resource may not sound like much of an endorsement, but for doulas to be acknowledged by the ACOG and SMFM as one of "the most effective tools" for improving labour and delivery outcomes is a significant professional recommendation. This statement reaffirms the importance of continuous support from professional doulas for improving outcomes for mothers and babies.

ETHNOGRAPHIC EVIDENCE OF DOULA SUPPORT

While the data in favour of doulas is clear, what remains unclear, or at least far less nuanced, is what specifically accounts for these improvements. Studies often cite doula support as providing increased mobility for the labouring woman, assistance with breathing or massage, and emotional support. Gruber, Cupito and Dobson, for example, have written that "constant presence" is a key aspect of doula work, and they state that doulas provide emotional support and "specific labor support techniques and strategies, encouraging laboring women and their families, and facilitating communication between mothers and medical caregivers" (50). Gilliland is more detailed and cites "specific labor support skills," "guidance and encouragement," covering "gaps" in care, "building a team relationship," and "encouraging communication" between the clients and the staff (762). In what follows, I critique previously published accounts of doulas and add to our understandings of the methods and strategies of experienced doulas as they describe their own birth work tools and tactics.

Bari Meltzer Norman and Barbara Katz Rothman argue that doulas may not actually make birth better; rather, they might just make women feel better about the (bad) births they have had (262). They critique doulas as "chameleons" (262) practised in passivity who try to help women without "ruffling feathers," questioning medical providers, challenging the medical model, or actually advocating for women (263). They argue that "doulas are women hired to be women, to demonstrate every conventional gendered tactic, strategy, stance, and emotion you can imagine" (251). Norman and Rothman note that doulas operate between medicine and mothers and have no real power (263). Because of this dynamic, they state that doulas have a tendency to "downplay themselves as professionals" by "playing dumb" (268) and being "like mimes" (269).

Norman and Rothman assert a primary distinction between doulas and midwives, calling doulas "experts in companionship" and midwives "birth experts" (279). Although they acknowledge that "women benefit from the presence of a supportive and knowledgeable labor companion," (255) Norman and Rothman question if this person need be a doula and suggest that doulas are women hired just to "put a supportive woman's body in the room with the laboring women" (259). Arguing that doulas need to take a clear stand on how birth should go rather than supporting mothers "without making some sort of political statement" (279), they conclude that "in trying to make quiet waves, doulas ultimately help along the current medicalized system of birth" (280) and, as such, might just be making women feel "good" about their "bad" births. Their conclusions, drawn from a limited study (253-254), do not account for the mounting medical data in favour of continuous labour support from trained doulas. The ethnographic research that I collected helps demonstrate why doulas improve outcomes for mothers and babies.

Norman and Rothman drew from a small and inexperienced pool of doulas in making their critique. Mindful of the importance of having experienced doulas with tenure in this profession speak to their work and shape our understandings of what doulas do,

I crafted my study with attention to representing the voices of established doulas from around the country. In February-March of 2014, I surveyed fifty-two doulas from thirty-one states, representing forty-four cities. Each doula had been working for more than three years (and most for closer to a decade) and all were trained and certified through a national or international certifying agency. Attendance at fifty births as a doula was the minimum requirement for participation, with a reported range of 53 to 845 births. The total number of births attended collectively from this sample set was 19,962. The average number of births attended was approximately 380, and the median experience level was about 150 births. All of the doulas responding had worked in private practice offering prenatal and postpartum visits for paying clients. About half of the doulas had also volunteered through various organizations and for different types of clients in need, such as military families, teenagers, homeless people, incarcerated women, and mentally disabled women.

I asked each doula how she accounted for the improved outcomes that studies have repeatedly linked to doula support. They responded to the question, "What, specifically, do you think you do with clients that increases the number of vaginal births, decreases the use of pain medication, and increases the APGARs of babies at birth?" Doulas repeatedly cited both prenatal counselling with clients and the unique perspective that they gain through continuous labour support as key to their positive impact on birth outcomes.

DOULA SUPPORT PRENATALLY:
"CHINESE FOOD AT A KOSHER DELI?"

Although doulas are usually hired for their expertise and support during labour and birth, they begin to help from the time that they are hired, often months before the birth. During pregnancy, doulas meet with clients to answer questions, assist with decision making, offer emotional support, and prepare for the birth and postpartum period. Doulas whom I interviewed identified a number of ways they help clients prenatally that they believe have a significant impact on their clients' birth outcomes. This prenatal assistance includes helping clients to feel calm and confident in pregnancy, helping clients see themselves and their bodies as capable, providing evidence-based information and educating clients about pregnancy and birth, assisting clients in articulating their preferences, facilitating their search for a care provider and birth location that matches their hopes and plans for the birth, and encouraging them to make the best possible decisions for themselves throughout their experience.

Doulas consistently reported that a key element of their work prenatally is to provide information and reassurance to help their clients stay calm and reduce their fear and anxiety about labour and birth. A doula who assisted at over 350 births reported:

> *A client recently told me that after meeting with me she went from feeling afraid of her upcoming birth to feeling excited about it. She had gained so much confidence through having her questions answered and knowing that she would have me there with her as a guide and for support. Even before labour had begun, I had already helped her transform her experience of birth.*

Another doula, with experience at over 550 births, articulated the importance of assisting with decision making prenatally:

> *Even before births I think I make a difference in these outcomes by redirecting them to providers more supportive of normal birth. I give a checklist of detailed questions for them to ask their doctors, so they know exactly what their doctors' practices are, so they know if they're trying to get Chinese food at a Kosher deli.*

This was a common response. Doulas repeatedly recognized the importance of helping direct clients to care providers who are more respectful, more evidence-based, and more likely to support the type of birth that the clients say they would like to have (Gilliland). Experienced doulas reported knowing the local playing field well and being able to help their clients find better medical care providers and/or better hospitals. Doula prenatal education and counselling encompass the first stage of improving birth outcomes, long before the labour has begun.

FRAGMENTED MEDICAL CARE AND THE "GLUE THAT HOLDS IT TOGETHER"

Continuous support is a central tenant of doula work, and in a fragmented health care system, doulas often cited this uninterrupted presence as a primary reason for improved outcomes. One doula wrote:

> *In our current compartmentalized birthing system, there is a huge need for the doula role. It is the glue that sticks the pieces of the experience together.... The most important thing that I think I bring to the team is consistency and continuity at hospitals. I see shifts change, and therefore I see care change (and sometimes dramatically). I see things missed.*

As an experienced doula who attended over 500 births, she likened her continuous labour support to reading an entire book; her attention to the emotional state and needs of her clients allows her to, "see more things." She wrote, "It's like reading every page in the book instead of just coming in for the 4th-10th chapters and expecting to understand the whole story. Noticing things is just a side effect of paying attention."

Similarly, a doula with experience at over two hundred births wrote:

> *Continuous care means that there is one person (the doula) that is taking ALL aspects of the labour into account and minding the collective impact this is having on the mom and her partner and her baby. No other person on the birth team comes to the table with this much perspective.*

This unbroken perspective, the "minding of the collective impact," is not a perspective that care providers and hospital staff get because they work in shifts and often with multiple labouring women at once. Furthermore, doulas provide support from much earlier in labour than medical providers routinely do, as evidenced by nearly every doula citing her support at home as a key tool for improving outcomes and experience. Even when women, as Gilliland states, are not medically "considered to be 'in labor' and do not qualify for hospital admittance," doulas are present supporting, comforting, and encouraging their clients (768).

One doula discussed in detail how her continuous presence can reduce the likelihood of Caesarean sections and improve outcomes for newborns. After over two hundred births, she shared this reflection: "Many times I have watched the patterns of the fetal heart rates and felt an intuition about the positions for mom because of this: positions that will keep the labour moving, keep the baby in optimal positioning and tolerating a long labour, better than if there was intermittent observation." This doula notes her unique access to the interaction between the labouring woman and her baby as she watches how the fetal heart tracing is affected by the mother's movements. Nurses and doctors usually watch a remote screen displaying the fetal heart tracing, but a continuously present doula can use this information to help the labour progress and keep the baby healthy. Another doula similarly referenced this perspective saying, "Continuous support in the room allows for the true continuous fetal tracing. I can move mama if baby shows decels or let a nurse know it was just mother moving and decrease false alarms." In this case, doulas serve as a bridge spanning hospital staff, the fallibility of technology, and the labouring mother.

Doulas can help to cover the gaps in modern maternity care (Gilliland 768), improving outcomes for her clients and their babies through continuous support. After attending over eight hundred births, one doula described her bridging role:

> Being in the room continuously I know where the frustration lies with the family. [I know] what they have tried in labour as far as positions or ideas [and] have known in advance what their goals are. I feel like I'm a bridge between that knowledge and the nursing staff who is in there minutes of every hour.

She described a scenario in which her bridging role might significantly change the outcomes: "A nurse might enter the room during a difficult contraction and feel like it would now be beneficial to administer medication—whereas the doula may know that this is an unusual contraction that the mom can get on top of and then proceed to another position or a cool cloth." She wrote that doulas are the only people who might see the "whole picture" in the room and, as such, offer an invaluable perspective.

BEING A WITNESS, OFFERING PERSPECTIVE, SLOWING THINGS DOWN

"I can not promise my clients a certain type of birth (like a vaginal birth versus a c-section), but I can promise them that they will not be alone, that I will help them in any way that I can, and that I will be a witness," one doula wrote. She clarified that she did not mean witness in the judicial sense (although that could also be true) but rather that the act of her being there with her clients is powerful in itself. The concept of being a witness powerfully references both the Christian Bible and the U.S. American civil rights movement, and for this doula it is a promise that she makes to all of her clients. In this role as witness, several doulas noted that their presence alone helps to improve the behaviour and decisions made by care providers and nurses. A doula with over four hundred births experience, for example, wrote, "I think being present encourages good behavior by the hospital staff and doctors." She suggests that being observed by an outside advocate might encourage care providers to give better care and behave more kindly.

Furthermore, doulas move between homes, birth centres, and different hospitals and work with a wide range of local care providers. This affords them a unique perspective on local maternity care. One doula referenced this by stating: "We are the only ones who get to step in and out of different hospitals and get to compare what actually happens in each delivery suite." She felt that doulas needed to remember the importance of their access to this wider perspective on maternity care. Another doula stated that after attending over 350 births she is able to give her clients access to the distinction between medically evidenced practices and non-evidence based hospital policies. She wrote, "I can help them see that there is nothing universal or prescribed about their treatment by a specific care provider or member of the hospital staff and that they can be treated differently in different places or by different care providers." She noted, for example, that she might be able to help a client understand how arbitrary a hospital rule can be by highlighting that another hospital a few miles away might have a completely different policy.

Having a doula present can be empowering for labouring women and their partners, helping them to be more assertive about their own care. A doula who had attended 150 births told me, "I've had many families say to me that just having me sitting with them in their room gave them the courage and confidence to speak up and ask their questions, ask for options, and ask for time to make decisions." By being an outside advocate, this doula suggests that her clients feel more confident in a medical environment where they might have otherwise have less capable of asserting themselves. Another doula wrote: "I help them find their voices and trust themselves as mothers and women. I help empower them to be strong and meet their goals whatever they are. This often means they find out they are stronger than they ever knew."

Doulas help women have better births by helping clients to find their voice, making space for asking questions, and assisting with informed choices. In our current highly medicalized and technology-driven maternity care model, so many healthy and low-risk women are being (over)treated and subjected to medical procedures and interventions with no proven benefit, and many with increased risks ("Choices" 2). Helping women to find their voice and to ask questions within this system allows true informed consent: women have the information and knowledge they need to make choices about their care. As educators and advocates, "doulas slow the process down," as one doula wrote. This slowing down was not about "making birth longer" but rather about "allowing families to have the time and space to collect the information they need to make the decisions that feel right to them." Because medical interventions can "snowball" and people can end up with "no idea how they got from one place to another in labour," one doula stated that her goal is to "slow down overwhelming situations" so parents have time to think and process their choices. These responses resonate with Gilliland's observation that doulas can help facilitate discussion, negotiation, and compromise as a bridge between mothers and care providers "often spanning different philosophies and perspectives about normal birth" (762).

BIRTH EXPERTS:
THE UNIQUE PERSPECTIVE OF CONTINUOUS CARE

Above I referenced Norman and Rothman's assertion that "there is a difference between an expert in birth and an expert in companion skills" (279). They argue that midwives are birth experts with "finely honed and trained companion skills" but question if doulas have any expertise (279) besides simply being women (251). I argue that doulas are experts in birth and that doulas' unique expertise accounts for the significant improvements evidenced in the medical literature. Doulas gain a distinct perspective by routinely attending more "entire labors from start to finish" (Gilliland 764) than other birth workers, by working in a wider variety of birthing institutions and with different care providers, and by attending to the hopes, fears, plans and goals of their clients. I argue that doulas improve birth outcomes for mothers and babies because of their emphasis on continuous care, and the unique expertise in birth that this continuous care teaches.

Speaking about her work, one doula described labour as "a journey and the doula is taking the steps alongside the mom." This process of taking steps alongside the mother is unique to doulas among birth workers. Although there are some care providers who practice this way, most obstetricians, midwives, and nurses do not. It is increasingly rare to find any birth professionals, other than doulas, present with labouring mothers throughout their entire journey. Furthermore, while care providers need to be attentive to their medical, legal, and institutional responsibilities, doulas are not bound to these in the same way and thus are free to be very physically and emotionally present with their clients. After attending over 250 births, one doula spoke about this presence: "I think being the one person in the room that is

100 percent connected to their emotional state makes the most difference. Smiling at them, encouraging them, honoring their sadness." This intimate connection with clients is often special to doulas and allows them to bring "humanity and care into the process." For another doula, her connection to the client and her presence throughout the experience allows her to make "individualized suggestions and not the one size fits all techniques that nurses and care providers give." It is the doula's intimate knowledge of this individual woman and her body, coupled with her knowledge of birth, that allows her to make individualized suggestions during labour.

This type of intimate connection and individualized suggestion making can result in improved outcomes when compared to taking a routine approach to treating complications in birth. One doula, for example, spoke of a recent birth when the baby was not coming under the pubic bone during pushing. The doctor was concerned and began "to discuss forceps and a possible cesarean." These routine suggestions were ultimately unnecessary after the doula assisted with a different pushing position, one that her experience with this woman during labour had led her to believe might work. In this new position, the baby came "under the pubic bone in one push." The doula said that the doctor was surprised and impressed after the birth and commented that she was able to achieve with position change what he had wanted to do with forceps or surgery. Another doula similarly described a birth where a midwife recommended pitocin to help labour progress, but the doula had seen the mother's contractions get stronger in an upright position, sitting nearer to her husband. The nurse encouraged the mother to lie in the bed separated from her husband by bed rails, which appeared to slow progress significantly. Rather than receiving pitocin, the doula helped the mother negotiate for more time and got her upright and in touch with her husband. This combination resulted in a vaginal birth without pictocin or other interventions. Both of these examples show how insights gained from continuous labour support allowed doulas to work with clients individually to improve their births and decrease unnecessary interventions.

Furthermore, the example above of the couple who laboured

best in close contact offers insights into how doulas can affect the biochemical well-being of labouring mothers and the hormones that encourage labour. Several doulas specifically referenced their support of labour hormones. One wrote, "Oxytocin is queen." She said that she helps women feel safe and loved so that their oxytocin levels stay high. Another doula wrote, "For the hormones of labour to flow freely, a woman needs to feel safe, secure, confident and have privacy." She said that a doula can be instrumental in creating this environment, especially in the hospital, a place that few people would describe as conducive to privacy and feelings of love and comfort. Turning down lights, getting extra pillows, playing music, helping a mother to be near her partner, building rapport with the nurses—all of this can help make a more intimate space for a birthing woman. Encouraging and praising her (and helping others to) can boost confidence. Offering massage or touch (and helping others to) can increase feelings of love and being cared for. This recognition of each woman's individual experience and how her body is best supported in birth is a very different perspective that doulas can bring to a medical model of childbirth.

In my study, doulas commonly spoke of techniques and tools they use to encourage optimal fetal positioning and to help mothers cope with labour without pain medication. They wrote about massage and counter-pressure techniques, the use of TENS machines (a transcutaneous electrical nerve stimulation device used to assist with pain), and rebozos and peanut and birth balls. They wrote about encouraging women to have showers and baths, keeping labouring women hydrated and nourished, offering emotional support and reducing fear, and increasing their clients' confidence in their own ability and strength. These techniques and tools were not employed in routine ways, rather doulas described "reading the body" and "watching the labour" to guide them in deciding when to use a different strategy most effectively. The cumulative impact of these forms of support, when employed by skilled doulas with the unique expertise learned through continuous care, account for the overwhelmingly positive body of data about doula supported birth.

Doulas are experts in birth and have an expertise that is largely unique to their training and practices. They seek to reduce fear and build confidence, increase knowledge and informed decision making, offer practical support for coping during labour and birth, and help preserve the memories of the birth story. Through counselling clients prenatally, supporting their search for care providers and birth locations that match their desires and needs, offering non-judgmental support continuously throughout labour, covering the gaps in modern maternity care, slowing the birth process down and serving as a bridge between labouring women and the hospital staff, offering individualized support and recommendations, and helping clients to cope with the physical and emotional challenges of labour—doulas improve births for both women and infants. Ethnographic evidence illuminates these specific methods, tactics, strategies, and practices cited by experienced doulas.

With maternal mortality rates rising, severe birth complications increasingly common, and a new reliance on technology and medical interventions that has not made women and their infants safer overall, we face a maternal health care crisis in the U.S. (Choices 1). More widespread access to doula care could significantly improve outcomes, yet doula support is vastly underused and sometimes resisted. I began this essay with the quote, "If a doula were a drug, it would be unethical not to use it" (DONA 1). Ironically, if a doula were a drug, it probably would be administered routinely, unlike the current status of doula care.

In this essay, I have shown a model of maternity care where doulas support women in finding their voice and their authority, where women are assumed to be capable and competent, and where labouring women are supported through non-medical inter- ventions such as massage, positioning, and encouragement. This non-medical care has been proven valuable in numerous studies and through my own ethnographic evidence, as illustrated above. Doulas improve births because of their unique emphasis on continuous care and the expertise gained from this continuous care. This critical information about doulas can help them gain the respect that they deserve for the unique expertise they bring to birth teams and for the valuable role they can play in turning the tide towards healthier mothers and babies in the U.S.

WORKS CITED

Choices in Childbirth. *Doula Care in* NYC: *Advancing the Goals of the Affordable Care Act.* New York: Choices in Childbirth. 2014. Print.

Davis-Floyd, Robbie. "The Technocratic, Humanistic, and Holistic Paradigms of Childbirth." *International Journal of Gynecology and Obstetrics* 75.1 (Nov. 2001, Supplement 1): S5-S23. Print.

Doulas of North America International. John H. Kennell, MD. DONA International Founder 1922-2013. DONA, 2013. Web. 16 June 2014.

Gaskin, Ina May. *Ina May's Guide to Childbirth.* New York: Bantam, 2003. Print.

Gilliland, A. "Beyond Holding Hands: the Modern Role of the Professional Doula." *Journal of Obstetrics, Gynecologic, & Neonatal Nursing* 31.6 (Nov-Dec 2002): 762-9. Print.

Gruber, Kenneth, Susan Cupito, and Christina Dobson. "Impact of Doulas on Healthy Birth Outcomes." *Journal of Perinatal Education* 21.1 (Winter 2013): 49-58. Print.

Gurevich, Rachel. *The Doula Advantage: Your Complete Guide to having an Empowered and Positive Birth with the Help of a Professional Childbirth Assistant.* New York: Prima Publishing, 2003. Print.

Hodnett, E., S. Gates, G. Hofmeyr, and C. Sakala. *Continuous Support for Women during Childbirth. Cochrane Database of Systematic Reviews.* 15 July 2013. Web. 12 May 2014.

Hwang, Suein. "As 'Doulas' Enter Delivery Rooms, Conflicts Arise." *The Wall Street Journal,* 19 Jan. 2004. Web. 9 June 2014.

Klaus, M., J. Kennell, and P. Klaus. *Mothering the Mother.* Boston: Addison-Wesley Publishing Company, 1993. Print.

Marshall H. Klaus, John Kennell, and Phyllis H. Klaus. *The Doula Book.* Third Edition. Cambridge, MA: Perseus Publishing, 2012. Print.

Martin, Emily. *The Woman in the Body: A Cultural Analysis of Reproduction.* Boston: Beacon, 1992. Print.

Morton, Christine and Clift, Elayne. *Birth Ambassadors: Doulas and the Re-Emergence of Woman-Supported Birth in America.* Amarillo, TX: Praeclarus Press, 2014. Print.

Paul, Pamela. "And the Doula Makes Four." *The New York Times*, 2 March 2008. Web. 9 June 2014.

Perez, Paulina and Snedeker, Cheryl. *Special Women: The Role of the Professional Labor Assistant*. Third Edition. Seattle: Pennypress, 2000. Print.

Scott, K. D., G. Berkowiz, and M. Klaus. "A Comparison of Intermittent and Continuous Support during Labor: A Meta-Analysis." *American Journal of Obstetrics and Gynecology* 180.5 (1999 May): 1054-9. Print.

2.
Retrieving the Maps to Motherhood

ALISON BASTIEN

HOW DOES A BODY KNOW to initiate labour? Whose body decides: the mother's or the baby's? Most of us may not think too often or too hard about these questions, but when you are expecting a baby—one that's come in and later will come out of your very own body—you may dimly realize that the new territory a new being must navigate to come into the world is *you*, via *your body*. Our current systems of childbirth preparation and doula trainings give women maps that focus on the known, carefully analyzing and charting all the outer choices to be made, as if they were the landmarks to be navigated. Culturally, we map choices about which tests to get when. We point women to the choice between hospital, birth centre, or midwife. We signpost epidurals or inductions, water birth or Caesarean, Ergo Baby or Moby Wrap, and cloth diapers or disposable ones. But we don't map the inner journey a woman and baby must make to give birth. In the clinical mapping of birth, the protagonist is the cervix—dilation and effacement tell us "where we are" in labour. The antagonist is time—as in *your water broke ten hours ago, you've been at four centimeters too long, your due date was five days ago, you're pushing too long. You're not even dilated. You're only six centimeters and it's been x hours, you're ten centimeters and it's not even coming!* As a midwife, doula, and childbirth educator, as well as trainer of midwives for nearly thirty years, I have come to believe that we need to "get on the same page" literally and start to share the same map, a map that details the inner journey as much more than the outer

32

one. This chapter focuses on how doulas can inadvertently get in the way of a mother's inner journey.

Midwife Diane Bartlett's research on brain waves helps provide the signposts for mapping the inner journey of birth. A woman in labour moves through four main brain wave states during the process of labour: 1) *beta brain waves*—those of the rational, note-taking and talking mind; 2) *alpha brain waves*—those of slight distraction but able to focus when needing to; 3) *theta brain waves*—those of the daydreaming or meditative state; and 4) *delta brain waves*—those of deep sleep or altered states of consciousness. Another way to understand this is to think that beta and alpha brain wave states reflect the forebrain or rational brain. Theta state reflects more the emotional or subconscious mind, and delta state takes us to the unconscious mind, the place where we are truly one with all that is. Mapping labour through these four different states paints a different picture of the landscape through which a labouring woman must journey.

In my work as a childbirth educator and trainer, I draw this map on the board for each group of students—be they pregnant couples, midwives, or doulas. The map takes the shape of a trip upriver in a kayak. In early labour, at the river's edge, we find the woman, her partner, and her doula, or other relatives excitedly documenting the beginning of her journey as the pregnant woman enters the kayak. She enters a single person kayak as only the mother can make this journey to bring forth her baby. The partner and others may be sloshing in the river alongside her or behind the kayak, giving it encouraging pushes, keeping her company, helping her get the feel of things as she navigates the river and its flows. The mother is still in the beta brain wave state, and in clinical terms we call this *prodromal* labour or early labour. Eventually, the well-wishers realize that the river's strong current is pulling the woman in her kayak along on its own. They also realize they are getting very wet and that the water is getting very deep, perhaps up to their chins, and their help is becoming less effective. They can feel the birthing woman pulling away into her own world. The clinical map would note cervical dilation now at nearly five centimeters and label her location as "entering active labour." I would mark her location as moving from alpha brain wave state into the dreamier theta state and map her location at the bend upriver, heading towards the big rocks. Alpha brain waves begin to let go of thoughts like: *how many centimeters? How much longer?*

At this point, the woman is moving inward to the theta state—characterized by longer, deeper breathing patterns—to meet the stronger contractions. Her gaze may move from focusing outward on the environment or her partner to an inward place where those around her are not able to go. The river on my map goes around a bend, and there the woman in her kayak discovers two huge boulders flanking the narrowing of the river. She hadn't seen this coming, and she realizes there is no turning back. She must pass through the dangerous looking gap between the boulders, even though she clearly hears a rushing waterfall beyond the bend. Clinically, this is active labour; a woman is six to eight centimeters dilated, getting close to transition. Transition is the powerful and chaotic place of eight to ten centimeters dilation. In my map, the fear of entering through the rocky pass and what it will entail represents transition. A woman on her inner journey who is uninterrupted and has no external interventions pressed on her enters into delta brain wave state during transition: a deep trance, removed from time and logic. In this state, she will take what time she needs to move past the rocks and waterfall, breathing deeply or seeming to be sleeping in between contractions, letting the waterfall take her. When she does this, she becomes fully open (ten centimeters) and experiences a deep calm. This is the calm prior to the expulsive phase, or fetal ejection reflex, as clinicians call it. Here, she finds herself no longer on the river but in a deep, still pool of water, where she rests and floats in her kayak, waiting for her baby to bob its head to the surface to indicate where it is and that it's ready for her to receive it. In the map I propose, the mother waits for the readiness of the baby to appear, not on the need to push simply because she is ten centimeters dilated.

Today, when a woman is looking to navigate her journey of labour into motherhood, she discovers that we have displaced the inner journey with a shopping trip. Culturally, we ask her to follow the path with a dozen certified professional guides—the prenatal yoga/dance/movement therapist, the childbirth educators, the prenatal doula, the doctor, midwife, ultrasound technician, birth doula, anesthesiologist, pediatrician, lactation specialist, and postpartum doula. They all have their own maps and guidelines for what is "normal" or "risky" for *their* part of the journey. They are not looking at the journey from the perspective of the mother. We frame the forks in the road in terms of "risk and pain management." Instead, we need to see the mother as receiving important information about what her body was made to do, knows how to do, and how she can best allow it to do so. And we leave her actual family out on the sidelines.

This is where my concern for doulas and other specialists on any given birth team comes into play. Doulas are often trained to be experts in using birth "accessories": the *rebozo,* the birthing ball, aromatherapy, massage tools, etc. But in my experience, these well-meaning interventions often keep the birthing woman from moving her focus inward and out of her rational mind to meet her baby and bring it through her body. The map for this journey is not outside. It is within each of us. Most doulas, in their enthusiasm and training, believe it is their caring and cheering and guidance that helps the woman get through birth. They miss the power of the labouring woman's inner journey. In many cases, the doula herself seeks healing and connection with the deeper feminine aspects of the mystery of birth; for many women witnessing and participating in this sacred journey of childbirth is profoundly restorative. Many doulas come to the profession because they have not experienced birth themselves and want to participate. Others are drawn to doula work to heal from a negative birth experience. Some doulas want to right a social wrong in how they perceive birthing women are treated in labour and birth. Some doulas want to test the waters to see if they want to train to become midwives or doctors later on, when their children are grown. Entering doula work for these reasons becomes problematic when they cast the doula as the central figure in the journey of birth.

Mothers may wish to hire doulas to act as a mother figure without having the "emotional baggage" of their actual mother. They want the support of someone who knows about these things. They want someone who is "clearly on their side" in the foreign territory of the medical setting. They set out with the map of the external clinical knowledge; the protagonist of their journey is the cervix, and its sidekick, time. This map never veers off course from the land of the beta brain waves and thus never leads the mother to where the baby really is waiting in delta state, where all of life emerges. The expectant mother thinks the doula has the map. In fact, most times, the doula hopes to *follow the mother* to her place of mystery and power by being with her at birth. If the doula holds out the clinical map with herself as the true guide, she will be offering a limited service to both the birthing woman and to herself because no standard map will get them where they are going. The doula inadvertently leads the birthing mother into a forest thick with all manner of professionals and protocols, and she is led further and further from the river that flows within herself towards her baby. This thick forest makes it difficult for the doula to find her bearings as well. The doula may feel frustrated and disempowered if the birthing woman makes choices the doula is not in agreement with. The doula may not see the options available in a vacuum of incomplete medical information, as she is not the caregiver nor is she allowed to make any medical assessments or offer any treatments. She may not direct the course of a chosen intervention either, except to the extent she can urge the labouring woman to do so. This urging bounces the labouring woman back into analytical beta state and hinders her journey. The doula also has the disadvantage of having to assess situations with very little emotional context to frame them in, and because doulas are not clinical experts, they take no responsibility for the outcomes in the moment or in the long term. Not only does she have incomplete autonomy in her own role at the birth but she also often supplants the potential for the actual family members to step up and find themselves in new levels of intimacy and responsibility with the birthing woman.

We become so full of our own competencies as caregivers that we may lose sight of who, in fact, is doing the actual work of labour. The success of a doula's work depends on her ability to let the woman go—to let her follow the map that leads deep inside her, not the clinical map that leads from one intervention to the other, or the map that sees labour as dodging interventions. Doulas often describe their work as "being present" for the woman in labour, but I even wonder in what ways "being present" hinders the *birthing woman* from being present for herself, her family, and her baby. When family or close friends are encouraged to learn and share in the journey from early in pregnancy, a doula may be redundant or even taking energy for her own healing on some level. Doulas also describe their role as bearing witness. Traditionally, a witness may be an important participant validating transitions in life. We have the witness at weddings, graduations, funerals, christenings, and other ceremonies that signify a change in our place in society or in ourselves. The role of witness becomes more challenging in the context of abuse, such as the mother who could not stop the alcoholic father from abusing the child or the classmate too afraid to call out the bully. In some instances, the doula as witness leaves the birthing family angry that she was not willing or able to stop an intervention, or a Caesarean section, or the baby from having a problem, or the mother from feeling terrible pain. Equally, at times, the doula herself is frustrated and angry she witnessed birthing policies or practices that she did not approve or outcomes she felt were preventable had she been able to act. In these cases, the doula becomes an enabler instead of a witness, and "being there" is not considered a virtue. When doulas view the map of birth as an exterior one that is not linked to the internal journey of the woman, they cannot serve mothers and babies.

At the end of birth, many fundamental questions need to be asked. Was the birthing woman able to make her journey? Did we honour the journey and try not to interrupt it with fear? Did we respect that the mother and baby were the ones making the journey and transitions here, not us? Did we engage the mother and baby in the decision making at all times, using their health, responses, and willingness to continue their journey as our guide? Was the mother the protagonist and not her cervix? Did timelessness replace the clock as the compass by which we navigated? When the labour is slowed or stopped, fear and pain dominate. We need to remember that darkness and seclusion are our traditional ways to go inwards, not a handful of helpful cheerleaders at the bedside, even if their words are kind. Words require that the mother stay in her rational mind. My goal as a midwife is to help the mother leave her mind and enter her body. We need to reframe the stories of birth from those of victimization, danger and strategies, back to stories of mystery, reverence, and journey. We need to promote the woman's strengths and skills innate in her body. We need to remember as women, we *are the maps* on this journey. And all people have taken the journey to get here as babies. Thus, we can all have confidence that the way is well known, we just need to refamiliarize ourselves with the lost maps. This is the skill that I would challenge the doula to hone—not her knowledge, her tricks, her passion, her outrage, or her love—but her willingness to share the map inward and let the woman go.

WORK CITED

Bartlett, Diane. "The Holistic Stages of Labor." *The Matrona* 17 January 2012. Web. 21 May 2015.

3.

A Doula for the Mother and the Self

Exploring the Intersection of
Birth and Body Culture

SARAH LEWIN

Remember this, for it is as true as true gets: Your body is not a lemon. You are not a machine. The Creator is not a careless mechanic... Even if it has not been your habit throughout your life so far, I recommend that you learn to think positively about your body.
> —Ina May Gaskin, *Guide to Childbirth*

THE CULTURAL NOISE AROUND BODY AND FOOD, imbued with *healthisms* and pervasive fat phobia, continues to grow louder. Current female body culture entrenches preoccupations with the thin ideal and body perfection, and this ideology permeates every facet of body experience. This culture not only directs how women feed, celebrate, criticize, care for and perceive their own and others' bodies, but also profoundly affects women's experience of pregnancy, birth, and the postpartum period. Birth is one intimate moment in a woman's body story; a story shaped by a life-long history with food, body size, culture, and identity. Body politics take on new meaning during pregnancy and birth as the pregnant body intersects with conflicting narratives of health, morality, beauty, weight, and, of course, motherhood.

Doulas and birth advocates support the belief that birth is an opportunity for women to reclaim their bodies in a unique way. The doula enters the birth space with the goal of helping a mother navigate labour and trust her body's innate ability to bring her baby into the world. As an advocate, the doula affirms that a mother's body is strong and should be trusted. The doula's support challenges, perhaps even attempts to rewrite, the dominant body narrative wherein women are disordered and powerless. Furthermore, the doula herself is also often steeped in the same body culture, creating a relationship between the doula's personal body story and the labouring mother's experiences. Identifying the language and ideologies that the doula brings to the birth within the greater cultural context of female body politics helps uncover all the intended and unintended effects of doula support, particularly how doulas contribute to conflicting narratives of birth and female embodiment.

In this paper, I explore how mothers and doulas negotiate the larger cultural ideologies surrounding weight and embodiment. Analyzing the language used by doulas and birth advocates, I examine the intersection of this support with dominant female body culture. To frame this discussion, I begin by briefly outlining current dialogues surrounding weight, health, and femininity. I emphasize problems with routine biomedical care of the pregnant body and the conflation of body size with notions of health. Following this framing, I explore the role that doulas play in both radically challenging and confirming women's disordered embodiment through language of female intuition and the notion of embodied knowledge. Finally, I end by questioning how opposing narratives of women's bodies intersect in the birth space and what meanings they hold for the greater body story of both the labouring woman and the doula.

The concepts and ideas I explore in this paper come from both my background in social work, with a specialty in facilitating dialogues around body image, and my training and work as a labour doula. I draw on my postgraduate psychoanalytic training focused on attachment, trauma, and social theories grounded in the spectrum of embodiment. I have previously conducted fieldwork, collecting and sharing oral narratives around body and identity. I have engaged in local and international doula communities through trainings, community events and networking, and social media. I draw from all of these experiences in what follows.

CULTURAL NOISE:
FAT PHOBIA, THE EXTERNAL GAZE, AND THE BABY BUMP

The female body is a political canvas; food, hunger, fatness, and thinness become metaphors for more complex communications and cultural battles (Bloom et al. 56). The dangers of eating disorders and negative body image have become mainstreamed dialogues, yet preoccupations with body perfection remain ever present and often disguised in the language of health. Public health discourse surrounding an "obesity epidemic" contribute to a moral panic surrounding fatness in America (LeBesco 73). The obsession with the thin body, along with the vilification of fatness, is a relatively new social phenomenon (Fraser 13). Health is a desired state, but it is also a prescribed state and an ideological position (Metzl 1). Women in particular must navigate a unique set of body criteria, which include the medicalization and moralization of fatness within the complex history of objectification and distorted notions of femininity (Orbach). Size discrimination targets people of size, but no body goes untouched by its effects within the greater culture. Popular culture unanimously agrees on the materiality of the healthy body as something within personal control, making thinness a moral pursuit. This moral pursuit is not uniform: factors such as race, ethnicity, sexuality, gender identity, and ability, among others, mediate women's body narratives. Yet the cultural preoccupation with weight and size is found throughout the literature on health and the practice of medicine. It becomes each individual's civic responsibility to perfect his or her body (LeBesco 156). The institutional and social ramifications of living in a body that does not abide by the dictated norms encourages a culture of fear around size diversity (Sobczak 48).

Given this body culture, it is no surprise that women often meet the emotional and physical fluctuations that mark pregnancy with ambivalence. Researchers have begun to document the ways in which female beauty ideals are navigated during pregnancy (Nash 25). By the time they become pregnant, many women have become hypervigilant of their food intake and body size. In *Birthing from Within,* England and Horowitz poignantly write, "Listening to your body in the kitchen sets the stage for listening to your body in labor" (22). Yet, for pregnant women, finding balance between honoring internal body experience within the greater cultural narrative of the pregnant body can present unique challenges.

The cultural dissonance around body and food renders honouring each individual's instinctual sense of the body nearly impossible (Sobczak 40).

In teasing apart lived body experience from image, Bloom et al., write "eating when hungry, stopping when full, and listening to all internal bodily cues are at least guides to establishing the possibility of a 'true body' self" (126). In other words, eating in line with hunger and satiety sets the foundation for living inside of the body. Although this might seem easy, many women enter pregnancy numb to the experience of feeling the body from the inside out. If one of the most essential body signals (hunger) is consistently ignored, what can be assumed about women's other instincts and visceral reactions?

The pregnant body, like the fat body, becomes public territory to comment on and monitor in the name of health (Nash 70). Although weight gain during pregnancy is typically a sign of progress and good health, current dialogues around weight contribute to strict body surveillance during pregnancy. Routine weigh-ins, prescriptions for low-fat or low-carb diets, and lengthy lists of restricted foods as well as continuous medical and social commentary on the size of the baby and the belly, and strict hospital policies that forbid eating and drinking during labour can all work to keep a woman fearful and distrustful of her body's instincts (Nash 134). Routine prenatal care is valuable, but what happens during those visits is often more cultural than medical and can act in direct conflict with cultivating the opportunity for deep listening to the body and its needs. Routine medical care often reinforces ideology around weight and food intake that ignores body diversity and relies on a one size fits all approach to all bodies (Bacon 2008). This is mirrored in routine prenatal care with prescriptive weight gain restrictions for pregnant women (IOM Report Brief). Although the Institute of Medicine stipulates that excessive maternal weight gain is a risk to both mother and baby and must be monitored closely, these recommendations must be considered within the greater cultural fear of fatness.

Extensive research documents the multiple biases and prejudices among health care providers against people of size, and the effects this bias has on clinical judgment and practices (Puhl and

Brownell 792). This is critical to consider when assessing best practices for women of size during pregnancy and general attitudes towards weight gain. Furthermore, the American Congress of Obstetricians and Gynecologists (ACOG) statement on obesity and pregnancy advocates for weight monitoring and counselling patients on appropriate weight management despite stating that said guidelines have "yet to translate into reduced rates of cesarean delivery or morbidity" (11). In other words, current approaches to weight management during pregnancy for women of size have not improved maternal outcomes. The medical institution continues to promote weight management tactics (code for weight loss through diet programs) that not only have been proven to be ineffective but also are shown to increase long-term weight gain (Gaesser 38). Even with this evidence, care providers are continually recommended to discuss weight management and nutrition with patients. Naturalized ideas of health and fatness are so intrinsic that it is imperative to divorce the two and look back at an individual's emotional and physical well-being separate from weight and body mass index (BMI).

Monitoring women's weight during pregnancy has become part of routine prenatal care; however, it is important to consider the "nocebo effect" (Buckley 44) of such persistent weight monitoring in a weight-obsessed culture. Weight is one piece of a much larger picture in assessing health. Other indicators such as eating and activity habits, dietary quality, self-esteem and body image as well as physiological measures such as blood pressure, cholesterol levels, and blood lipids are argued to be more important pieces in assessing health (Bacon and Aphramor 2). It is essential to acknowledge the complicated and size-ist attitudes that women, health care providers, and doulas bring to the birth space, and how these prejudices become entrenched in routine prenatal care. Rarely is the emotional and physical harm and stress of this type of body monitoring considered. Continuous commentary on weight change for the mother, as well as predicted size of the baby, encourages a woman to unleash a critical voice, telling her that her body is flawed, and she cannot correctly grow and nurture her baby. These practices also highlight the inconsistent use of evidence-based research in routine prenatal care protocols regarding size of the baby and health outcomes (ACOG 13). Fears around weight of the baby and mother often speak more to larger cultural anxieties around size than to evidence-based medicine (McLellan 16). With fat phobia embedded in modern prenatal care, it is imperative for doulas to be aware of their own body history, and how it might affect the mothers that they support.

THE BIRTH SPACE:
THE DOULA, BODY STORIES, AND LANGUAGE

The birth space is a microcosm of the greater culture at large, and the practices and language surrounding it are riddled with double binds and social contradictions. The doula enters the birth space coming from the same body culture as the mother that she supports. In an effort to counteract negative societal messages about women's bodies and birth, many doulas encourage laboring women to trust their intuition. The language doulas use can unintentionally perpetuate a falsely nostalgic narrative of women's bodies as sacred. As the doula reminds the mother that her body is strong and intuitive, it must be assumed on some level that she is grappling with these notions herself, in her own body.

During the prenatal period, doulas frequently become sounding boards for pregnant women who receive, and already carry, internalized body criticisms regarding weight gain and baby's size; this often includes strict dietary changes recommended by doctors, often with little explanation as to why. Doulas are in a unique position as they can create more space for a mother to start exploring how that information sits within her unique body story. In order to do so, the doula must navigate her own culturally specific body ideologies and be cognizant of how her personal body story may be filtering the support that she is providing. In my experience working within the doula community, there still exists a tension between body trust and the cultural preoccupation with body size. This tension comes up casually and often unrecognized among doulas. I have seen conversations seamlessly go between empowering clients to trust their bodies to offhand statements about a doula's own belly size or weight-loss goals without any critical attention to these tensions.

Online doula communities are a rich public space for exploring how the culture permeates the support that doulas provide for their clients. Examples of how this manifests within the doula community can be seen on the Doulas of North America (DONA) Facebook group, a popular resource for doulas to post comments, ask questions, and connect with others. One doula posted that she was "shocked" to hear that one of her clients—who is in good health (normal blood pressure and no health concerns throughout the pregnancy) and entering her last trimester—had been bullied by her health care providers because of her weight (18 Jan. 2015). The doula's surprise that her client would be bullied for her weight speaks to the doula's own body experience, which has likely not included overt weight discrimination. The responses to her post ranged from echoing the doula philosophy of "her body is not broken and it knows just what to do" to doulas expressing concerns about the serious health risks associated with obesity. One doula, for example, wrote that this would be a "good opportunity to have her do a diet log and guide with nutrition" and stated that the client might have been "sensitive" and may have chosen to "be offended rather than maximize the situation while there is time to do so with ... diet, education, and exercise" (18 Jan. 2015). Interestingly, not a single doula responded to this post by stating that recommending a client to keep a food log and increase exercise was out of a doula's scope of practice. This recommendation—so readily accessible for this doula and yet clearly outside of DONA's scope of practice— demonstrates the greater cultural blind spot to issues around weight.

Conflation with weight and health is so strongly entangled that despite the original post explicitly stating that this mother was in good health, doulas primarily called on the use of empowering language to encourage this client or warned about the complications of obesity, and they suggested ways to help the mother adopt the doctor's feedback. It is not surprising that despite a strong consensus among doulas that a woman should not be shamed around her body by doctors, ambivalence continues to exist around how to help a mother navigate issues relating to body size. Directing clients towards evidence-based research is a linchpin of modern doula philosophy, and yet it is common in conversations between doulas to hear such evidence ignored in favor of repeating an ill-supported, yet constantly perpetuated caveat, that a mother may be in general good health, but we must never let her, or ourselves, forget that obesity is a serious danger.

In dialogues about body size, many doulas offer words of encouragement that rely on language of empowerment such as, "remind her that her body is not broken" and "it [her body] knows just what to do" (Facebook 18 Jan. 2015). Yet how does the encouragement of a doula counter the institutional forces that keep women doubtful of their bodies? The greater culture, including doctors, bombards a woman of size with daily reminders that her body is wrong or broken. Furthermore, when doulas themselves talk about supporting "plus-sized women," examples of their own bias creep in. In another DONA Facebook thread, for example, one doula wrote that heavier clients have a harder time staying on their feet during labour and suggested that doulas use a birth ball or rocking chair to support fat clients (25 Jan. 2015). A second doula affirmed this statement suggesting heavier clients would do well spending more time "in sitting and lounging type positions ... anything that will let mom move but not have to get exhausted from her own body weight" (25 Jan. 2015). Although it is possible that any client could become easily fatigued on her feet during labour, the assumption that supporting larger women during labour requires more time spent "sitting and lounging" is reflective of cultural narratives about fatness. These comments are mixed in with other doulas who say that they are "quick to reassure moms that show self-consciousness about their bodies that their bodies are amazing, beautiful, and strong" (Facebook 22 Jan. 2015).

These contradictory dialogues that doulas have about labour support and fat bodies point to the importance of continuing to analyze assumptions conflating health and weight to better support mothers of all sizes. These Facebook posts are just one example of how the language that doulas use around advocacy and empowerment are also imbued with unintentional moralizing and culturally biased attitudes towards weight and health. Doulas champion the idea that women are powerful and magical in their physical abilities to birth, yet many of them have histories of being doubtful of their own bodies, and this can affect the support a doula offers.

Interestingly, many doulas with whom I have spoken identify doula work as having helped them feel more positive about their own body. This was affirmed by a doula on Facebook who wrote, "I think my body image has improved as I see all shapes and sizes doing the most womanly thing possible" (22 Jan. 2015). In the process of witnessing women do the hard work of labour and reminding them they are strong, doulas are uniquely situated to challenge the dominant cultural narrative around female bodies. The experience of being a doula is partially about the production of this counter-narrative; when doulas tell their clients "you are beautiful and strong," on some level they must feel that themselves as fellow women. It is essential, therefore, to give doulas a larger framework for reflecting on their interaction with this counter-narrative, and the ways in which they engage with their body histories in the birth space.

Doulas learn through their training that birth support often occurs on a bodily level (i.e., massage, safe touch, being a continuous presence), but language is an important and underexplored component of this work. Women trust doulas not only with the intimate experience of childbirth but also with their naked bodies during a vulnerable time. How doulas engage their clients in dialogues about this experience prenatally, during the birth, and in the postpartum period is critically important for building trust and affirming a woman's body narrative. The language used by doulas typically situates itself within ideologies of the natural birth movement (despite the reality that most doulas attend births in highly interventionist hospitals) and draws heavily on affirmations of women's bodies as powerful, capable, and strong. Phrases such as "let your body tell you what to do," "you are so strong—strong enough for this," and "trust that you can do it," are examples of the language that doulas are taught to encourage labouring women (McGrath). For some women, these prompts may be empowering and may inspire a new-found body confidence. For others, however, this language can be alienating as it may be incongruent with that woman's lifelong experience in her body.

For the woman who may not have an understanding of what it means to trust her body, doulas need to go beyond one-dimensional scripts about intuition and trust. These prompts might be overwhelming rather than reassuring and keep a woman stuck in her thoughts instead of helping her fully inhabit her body during pregnancy and birth. Doulas can begin this language shift prenatally by exploring times when the woman has felt fully embodied and what that might have been like for her. From here, a doula can begin to gauge the comfort level that the woman feels and perhaps make space for discussing anxieties or fears about losing control during pregnancy and birth. This prenatal dialogue can set a stronger foundation for knowing the woman's body history and her potential needs during birth. This woman might need a different type of supportive language that strays from the scripts doulas are given, which naturalize women's innate wisdom. One example of an alternate type of support would be to focus on smaller steps that help her body release tension, such as "let's together take a deep breath in and then sigh out." After doing this with her a couple of times, the doula might say, "look at how your shoulders release tension and become heavy with each exhale. Your body knows how to regulate itself without you even having to think about telling it what to do." Showing a woman how the body has intuition rather than telling her can be a less threatening way to support a woman beginning to explore her body's intuitive responses. In the postpartum period, it is important to process this component of the birth by asking the mother what it was like to feel her body regulate itself in this way and explore the experience of listening to the body and its needs.

Doulas are not routinely trained to unpack their own bias and body history as it relates to size and health, so they may struggle to offer valuable support to their clients in the face of the overwhelming cultural noise around food and body size. Doulas are trained to consider structural inequalities within the maternity care system and are given tools to provide culturally sensitive birth support. Issues around weight, health and size, however, are not included in their training. As shown by the casual fat phobia in the online forum above, there is little or no formal training on size diversity or on how to support pregnant women negotiate issues around body and weight. In my experience engaging with doulas on this topic, there is a tendency to want to divert the attention onto their clients' experience rather than unpack their own personal body story and subsequent biases and assumptions. Doulas would benefit from having a chance to deconstruct their own body narrative in order to develop tools for supporting clients throughout their pregnancy. From here, the doula can authentically be present for the mother wherever she is in her body narrative and can acknowledge the greater cultural landscape that permeates every facet of the body self.

CONCLUSION: YOUR BODY IS NOT A LEMON!

Ina May Gaskin wrote, "No matter how much pressure our society may bring upon us to pretend otherwise, pregnancy, labor, and birth produce very powerful changes in women's bodies, psyches, and lives." She continues, "the journey through pregnancy and birth offers an irreplaceable way for women to explore their deepest selves—their minds, bodies, and nature" (*Birth Matters* 1). Many doulas hold this sentiment: the journey through birth and into motherhood has the potential to inspire a rewriting of one's body narrative. Given that notions of disorder and inadequacy communicated today through fatness and thinness dominate many women's narratives, a supported birth experience has the potential to challenge assumptions about what the female body can or cannot do. In this way, the support of the doula, along with the language of intuition and trust, is radical in a culture that conditions women to numb their appetite and desires through diets and healthisms.

The relationship between doula and mother is symbiotic, and their stories are intimately connected. As the doula supports the mother, the mother indirectly supports the doula by giving her the opportunity to advocate for female embodiment and agency. The doula has the potential to make a bridge for women who experience cultural objectification and alienation from their bodies to walk across, and while they will still be faced with the negative messages on the other side, they may begin to shift their understandings of their own bodies. As doulas cultivate awareness of the ideologies that silence embodied knowledge, they can become keenly aware of their personal assumptions and prejudices that emerge from their body narrative and the greater culture. The work of being embodied, intuitive and nurturing—all adjectives doulas use to encourage their clients during birth—must be turned to the self. From here, there can be more space within the doula-mother relationship for dialogues around the body history that each woman brings to the birth space and, subsequently, into motherhood.

Acknowledgements: I wish to express deep appreciation to Megan Davidson for her mentorship and insightful feedback on this chapter. I am also very grateful to Jillian Buckley for her thoughtful and important edits.

WORKS CITED

American Congress of Obstetricians and Gynecologists (ACOG). "Safe Prevention of the Primary Cesarean Delivery." Society for Maternal-Fetal Medicine, March 2014. Web. 28 Dec. 2014.

Bacon, Linda. *Health At Every Size: The Surprising Truth About Your Weight.* Dallas: BenBella Books, Inc, 2008. Print.

Bacon, Linda and Lucy Aphramor. "Weight Science: Evaluating the Evidence for a Paradigm Shift." *Nutrition Journal* 10.9 (2011): n.pag. Web. 3 Dec 2014.

Bloom, et al. *Eating Problems: A Feminist Psychoanalytic Treatment Model.* New York: BasicBooks, 1994. Print.

Buckley, Sarah. *Gentle Birth, Gentle Mothering.* New York: Celestian Arts, 2009. Print.

Fraser, Laura. "The Inner Corset: A Brief History of Fat in the United States." *The Fat Studies Reader.* Eds. Esther Rothblum and Sondra Solovay. New York: New York University Press, 2009. 15-23. Print.

Gaskin, Ina May. *Guide to Childbirth.* New York: Bantam Book, 2003. Print.

Gaskin, Ina May. *Birth Matters.* New York: Seven Stories Press, 2011. Print.

Gaesser, Glenn. "Is 'Permanent Weight Loss' an Oxymoron? The Statistics on Weight Loss and the National Weight Control

Registry." *The Fat Studies Reader.* Ed. Esther Rothblum and Sondra Solovay. New York: New York University Press, 2009. 37-41. Print.

Institute of Medicine. "Weight Gain During Pregnancy: Reexamining the Guidelines." *Report Brief.* 2009. Web. 28 Dec. 2014.

LeBesco, Kathleen. "Fat Panic and the New Morality." *Against Health.* Eds. Jonathan M. Metzl and Anna Kirkland. New York: New York University Press, 2010. 72-83. Print.

McGrath, Kathy. "Encouraging & Empowering Statements." *DONA International Training Packet,* 2008. Print.

Nash, Meredith. *Making 'Postmodern' Mothers: Pregnant Embodiment, Baby Bumps and Body Image.* London: Palgrave Macmillan, 2012. Print.

NcLellan, Jen. "Empowering Women of Size." *International Doula* 22.2 (2014):15-19. Print.

Metzl, Jonathan. "Introduction: Why 'Against Health'?" *Against Health.* Eds. Jonathan M. Metzl and Anna Kirkland. New York: New York University Press, 2010. 1-14. Print.

Orbach, Susie. *Fat is a Feminist Issue II.* London: Arrow Books, 1998. Print.

Post. *Facebook.* DONA International, 18 Jan. 2015. Web. 19 Jan 2015.

Post. *Facebook.* DONA International, 18 Jan. 2015. Web. 24 Jan 2015.

Post. *Facebook.* DONA International, 25 Jan 2015. Web. 1 Feb 2015.

Puhl, Rebecca and Kelly Browne. "Bias, Discrimination, and Obesity." *Obesity Research* 9.12 (2001): 788-805. Print.

Sobczak, Connie. *Embody: Learning to Love Your Unique Body (and Quiet That Critical Voice!).* California: Gurze Books, 2014. Print.

4.

"Screw You Guys! I'm Not a Bad Person"

Disrupting the Damaged Birthmother Model with Doula Support

SUSANNA C. SNYDER

To live in this world you must be able to do three things: to love what is mortal; to hold it against your bones knowing your own life depends on it; and, when the time comes to let it go, to let it go.
—Mary Oliver, "In Blackwater Woods"

DESPITE THE INCREASING VISIBILITY of adoption in the U.S., birthmothers, women who relinquish children for adoption, remain largely hidden. Birthparents are the "least understood and most-stigmatized participants in the [adoption] process," and, in lieu of personal contact or an accurate depiction in popular media, birthmothers are imagined within existing cultural scripts (Donaldson Adoption Inst *Safeguarding* 4). Most people imagine that to relinquish is to experience a loss. Although letting go of that you have held "against your bones," is certainly difficult, this characterization is one dimensional (Oliver n.p.). The birthmother in this narrow narrative is either trouble or troubled.

This chapter complicates that birthmother. The empowered experiences of doula-supported birthmothers can challenge the popular belief that birthmothers are damaged by the act of relinquishing. The ability of society and scholars to understand the experiences of these women has been limited by what I call the "damaged birthmother model"—the assumed pathology of a woman who chooses to biologically parent but eschews social parenting. I argue that this model does not reflect a "natural" reality; it has not necessarily been produced by a biologico-maternal imperative to parent and, thus, grieve the loss of the opportunity to parent (Leon *Losses* 125). Rather, this facile model that has dominated research and sentiment on birthmothers may reflect the stigma associated with a woman who "unbecomes a mother" (Gustafson 1; Wegar 77). Doula-supported birthmothers, myself included, who report feelings of empowerment associated with relinquishment, represent a counter-voice to this model. To that end, I examine the way doula support provides one avenue for birthmothers to resist the dominant cultural portrayal.

Research shows that social support improves physical, emotional and social health outcomes (Heaney and Israel 195). Additionally, literature on birthmothers has suggested that social support may mitigate the grief of relinquishment (Winkler and van Keppel 64). In providing specialized social support amid the choice to place a child for adoption, doulas are uniquely suited to help birthmothers realize a sense of empowerment in relinquishment. Although this research is not designed to prove causality between doula support and birthmother empowerment, the doula-supported voices heard here and the damaged birthmother narratives heard elsewhere stand in stark contrast to each other. The provision of doulas for birthmothers has the potential to improve not only the physiological outcomes of labour and delivery but also a birthmother's post-relinquishment readjustment. The research presented in this chapter supports this hypothesis and is intended to provide a foundation for future studies on doulas for birthmothers—a critical site of intervention for this largely hidden and poorly understood population.

POSITIONALITY AND METHODS

As a seventeen-year-old senior in high school, I spent a warm winter horrified and dazed by the knowledge that I was pregnant. Being white and middle upper class, I could have chosen to parent with the help of my family, and, being liberal and feminist, I could have terminated with the belief that it was my right. Yet, as the winter turned into spring, I chose to relinquish. I felt privileged to have been given those three choices, and profoundly changed by the one that I made. The pregnancy not only interrupted my adolescence, it also interrupted a cycle of self-destruction. Caring for myself, if even for the sake of the fetus inside of me, taught me a level of self-care and love that I had previously lacked. At the time, I imagined a healthy pregnancy and un-medicated vaginal birth as a gift to the coming baby, but the experience also became a gift for me. With the help of a doula, I found power in my pregnancy and relinquishment birth. Emerging on the other side of the adoption process, I was grieving yet more confidently grounded in my body and, ultimately, self—both were apparently far more powerful than I had previously assumed.

So, imagine my shock when I engaged the birthmother literature as a graduate student in anthropology. I was horrified to read the effects of relinquishment:

> depression, damaged self-esteem, persistent guilt, shame, and self-loathing over "giving away their child;" persistent loneliness or sadness; difficulty with intimacy, attachment or emotional closeness; lack of trust; anger; severe headaches or physical illness that cannot be expressed or diagnosed; and occasionally PTSD characterized by extreme anxiety, panic attacks, flashbacks and nightmares. (Fessler 211)

I began to feel depressed just reading about all the reasons that I was supposed to be depressed. This early literature on birthmothers had been groundbreaking. The women whose experiences had produced this research had relinquished in a time when accessible and effective birth control was the whisper of a dream, abortions were nightmarish back-alley affairs, and out-of-wedlock pregnancies were fodder for permanent pariah-hood (Melosh 132, 152, 19). Birthmothers of emerging generations may still be victims of restrictive reproductive health laws that allow the refusal of the morning after pill or victims of the sexism manifested in "illegitimate rapes," but their level of agency and potential for myriad outcomes has been altered by dramatic cultural and legal shifts (Donaldson Adoption Inst *Safeguarding* 6; Pertman 22).

The stark contrast between my experience and that reflected in the literature led me to ask: can a new generation of birthmothers, even when in a place of financial or emotional desperation, begin to realize some sense of self and sense of power in relinquishment? I evaluated the sources of strength in my relinquishment. At the onset of this research, I was still only beginning to understand the class and race privilege that allowed me this "choice" at all, so this research lacks the scope to evaluate the influence of these privileges. Instead, the use of a doula and her influence on my empowering birth experience led me to wonder: could other women making a plan of adoption realize similar benefits from having a doula?

To answer this question, I recruited three doula-supported birthmothers in a Midwestern state. They ranged in age from eighteen to twenty-two, had relinquished in the previous three years, and all identified as white and working class. They had all relinquished their first child and had completed high school. In interviews, I used a targeted life history approach, asking my participants to narrate their story from conception to present day, and followed up with semi-structured, open-ended questions (Schensul et al. 138; Ulin 64). Finally, I concluded each interview by encouraging participants to ask *me* questions about my experience since, during recruitment, two of the three participants commented on not having met a birthmother who had relinquished so long ago. Although I originally imagined this as a "give back" portion of the interview, this more reciprocal dialogue proved to be a rich site of data. I realized how embedded I was in this research, and what a gift this research was for me in my own emotional process (Rapp 14).

The results of these interviews show that in many areas, like social stigma and ambivalent motherhood identity, the participants report similar experiences to birthmothers in other studies, but the reports of empowerment stand in stark contrast to the majority of birthmother literature. An analysis of these findings requires a review of literature on adoption perceptions, birthmother needs, and the opportunity for doula support.

BACKGROUND

In the U.S. and other pronatalist societies, biological realities of reproduction have been elevated as social imperatives for gendered behaviour (Gustafson 1). For motherhood, this has generally meant

that the female body is assumed to be most fully realized in reproduction and parenting (Foucault 104; Ellison 323). Disciplinary
discourses of gender and kinship have maintained the notion
that maternity is not only a biological inevitability but it is also
a "civic duty" (Ellison 325). To decouple the reproduction from
the parenting, to "[unbecome] a mother ... is variously regarded
as unnatural, improper, even contemptible" (Gustafson 1).

This belief in the "damaged birthmother" is illustrated in public
sentiment, media depictions, and even the academic literature. A
national representative sample of adoption beliefs in the U.S. shows
that "Americans are divided over whether it is better for pregnant
teenagers to place their babies for adoption or raise them themselves," and, although the majority of the U.S. population supports
birthparents' decisions, one in four disapproves and feels that this
decision is irresponsible, uncaring, and selfish (Donaldson Adoption
Inst *Benchmark* ii). Although a stark minority, the power of a quarter
of the population to make one feel like a deviant is still very real. In
popular media, Amanda Karel analyzed 292 news stories covering
adoption and found similar results with more "problematic than
positive depictions," and, when birthparents were depicted (only
47 percent of the time), they were portrayed as "solely negative"
over twice as much as "solely positive" (492). Also, the negative
stories often focused on sensationalized stories about birthparent
reclamation—a statistically rare occurrence (Donaldson Adoption
Inst *Attitudes* 4). Biases against adoption are also found in and
perpetuated by academic sources. Content analysis of textbooks in
family research found that "little attention was devoted to adoption and that the coverage provided was predominately negative,
stressing the potential problems of adoption about twice as often
as its probable successes and rewards" (Fisher 154).

Birthmothers report an awareness of this stigma. Numerous
studies recount how birthmothers cannot express their feelings
of grief because they feel their experiences are shrouded in a
"conspiracy of silence" (Mander 131; Winkler and van Keppel
4; DeSimone 71; Logan 618; Brodzinsky and Smith 178). Aloi
employs Doka's concept of *disenfranchised grief* to categorize this
phenomenon and its impacts on birthmothers (27). Disenfranchised grief is "grief that is not openly acknowledged, socially

accepted or publicly mourned"—all of which mark the birth-mother experience (qtd. in Aloi 27). The effect is to intensify the grief, prolong its duration, and make the individual vulnerable to further losses (Aloi 29). Winkler and van Keppel found that the strongest indicator for maladjustment post-relinquishment was a lack of social support, described as an inability to "talk through feelings about relinquishment" (1). One birthmother stated this feeling well saying, "It is like somebody's died but when somebody dies it is different because it is talked about" (Mander 63). Over 78 percent of the birthmothers in the Winkler and van Keppel study wanted to discuss their feelings regarding their relinquishment. Those who reported that they could discuss their feelings exhibited a more satisfactory adjustment within twelve months postpartum (49).

Less literature explores the intrapartum care provided for birthmothers, but it merits review since the birth of the child and the act of separation both generally occur within the biomedical birth system. Leon argues that physicians are ill prepared to handle the special circumstances of relinquishment and must become better equipped (*Caregiver* 125); Mander makes a similar argument with midwives in the British model of care (179), and several articles (Aloi 30; Bond et al. 156; Devaney and Lavery 375) discuss the potential role of labour and delivery nurses in providing social support to mothers but note the difficulty because of busy labour and delivery wards. The birth experience for birthmothers is understandably bittersweet and difficult and could benefit from having a good labour experience. Devaney and Lavery found that "after exploring their feelings, most [birthmothers] want their birth experience to be as rewarding and emotionally fulfilling as that of married women" (377), but Mander found that "majority of relinquishing mothers [in her study] were not at all satisfied with their maternity care" (179). Unfortunately, because of low social and economic capital, lack of social support, and the absence of childbirth education, these women may enter the hospital with little to no knowledge of the childbirth experience and may be susceptible to feelings of being overwhelmed, isolated and not in control of their birth experiences (Devaney and Lavery 376).

Doulas are well poised to respond to these problems. Numerous studies have shown the quantitative (reduced Caesarean section rates, decreased length of labour) and qualitative (increased satisfaction with labour experience) impacts of doulas (Hodnett et al. 13). Other studies have shown the potential for additional benefits of doulas in vulnerable populations such as increased high school graduation rates for doula-supported teens and breastfeeding success for high-risk moms served by community-based doulas (Healthy Baby Project, "The Teen Parent Empowerment Project"; Health Connect One, "Perinatal Revolution"). These long-term psychosocial impacts are argued to be the result of an adage: "if you birth from a position of power, you can parent from a position of power" (Everson np). This research asks: if a birthmother births from a position of power, with the assistance of a doula, can she then *relinquish* from a position of power? The preliminary data presented here suggests that she can.

FINDINGS:
THE MISSING PIECES OF THE BIRTHMOTHER EXPERIENCE

After a year of literature review and grant writing, I walked into my participant interviews prepared to hear stories of intense grief that segued into depression and anxiety. Instead, my participants were bright-eyed women with multidimensional experiences that reflected the dynamism of love and loss. Their heart-wrenching accounts of letting go knotted my stomach in nostalgic knowing, but I was also drawn into the transformative narratives present in each story.

Although I do not want to diminish the grief in their stories or my own, I know that most readers have experienced some personal loss and can apply it to the stories of birthmothers—the script has already provided the story of birthmother loss. What that script is missing is an assessment of how a birthmother is affected by *being told* she will experience a loss that will cause irreparable harm, and how a birthmother may defy that script by feeling positively affected by relinquishment. I want to illustrate several critical points regarding birthmothers: first, how birthmothers are stigmatized by the choice to relinquish; second, how they respond to this stigmatization by resisting disclosure and increasing isolation; and third, how a support person, such as a doula, can help them through this loss by giving them tools to empower themselves in their relinquishment.

Stigma

For the women whom I talked to, close family members tended to be supportive, but community members and casual acquaintances passed painful judgment. Vicki (all participants provided pseudonyms), a 20-year-old woman who had relinquished five months prior to our interview, was told by her co-workers who had chosen to parent that she was a "bad mom" and that it "didn't matter what your living situation was," you don't "give up" a baby. Comments like these motivated Vicki to stop disclosing her birthmother status once she realized that, as she put it: "No one looks at you like, 'Oh, you really love this baby, that's why you're giving him a good family. Go you!'" She was the participant who reported the sentiment: "Screw you guys, I'm not a bad person."

Laura, who had relinquished at nineteen years old, experienced a large amount of stigmatization while she was pregnant and obviously unmarried, which caused her to buy herself a wedding ring. She also reported a variety of stigmatizing events because of her relinquishment. A more dramatic instance occurred when a man who had a negative adoption experience yelled at her: "You'll never ever see your baby again. They say that it's going to be an open adoption. But they'll back out on you. That's how it always works. You think you know how all of this works, well, let me tell *you*." Elizabeth relinquished at seventeen years old, almost a year before our interview. She was still navigating the choice to disclose amid experiences of feeling judged. She said, "I just need to be open with it and tell everyone that I have a baby and he's still in my life." But, she countered, "It's definitely a turn-off for people ... they just leave. They don't care to know what happened ... you must be a slut."

Empowerment

Despite these negative social experiences, these women also reported feelings of empowerment. Vicki, less than six months post-relinquishment, still struggled with the decision to relinquish, but regarding her pregnancy she said:

In a way, I loved being pregnant. It was so cool ... the first months when you can feel him moving around in there ... And the birth itself. Going into labour.... It wasn't fun for a lot, but the whole experience is just crazy. The whole fact that you have a human in there. Growing inside you. And then BAM there he is.... Such an awesome experience.... It was really cool. I'm kind of excited when, you know, the time is right. I can't wait to be pregnant again. I can't wait to do it again. It was fun.

Laura reported a similar awe with her birth experience: "I definitely have to say that my birth experience was awesome." She went into her birth incredibly informed and felt it was important that she undergo the process naturally, for her and the baby. She also described herself as a pushover prior to her pregnancy, "the little fighter for everyone but myself," but her narrative revealed that she very much advocated for herself and the baby. She reported that this was "out of character" but easier during pregnancy because she felt, "this is my baby and this is my body, and I am going to be making her into a child."

Elizabeth reported a significant increase in self-respect because of relinquishing but not the birth experience. For her, the major growth and transformation came after the birth when she held her son and met the adoptive family, a relationship that has developed into a deep friendship. Before becoming pregnant, she reported that she "was just naïve" and turned to the birthfather, her longtime boyfriend, for "closure" from her parents' divorce and struggled growing up without a strong maternal figure. Her growth was apparent in her reflection:

I think that this whole thing saved me.... I should have found something that I really enjoyed in life. And I looked to one thing, but it wasn't the best thing. Now, I have such a good outlook on life. It's not just about one person. You have to go out there and find what you love and be happy with what you do.... You have to broaden your focus. I don't think that other people should make me happy. I should be happy with what I do in life and stuff.

Also, all of the participants reported wanting to go into helping, birth-related professions as a result of their birth and/or relinquishing experience. Vicki wanted to be an ultrasound technician and was considering becoming a doula. Elizabeth had always been interested in a career in health but wanted to focus that work in a neonatal unit. Finally, Laura stated it most clearly, "because my birth experience was so awesome, that's what made me want to be a nurse-midwife. I want to provide that for someone else." Choosing careers that allow birthmothers to use their experiences of placing a child for adoption in meaningful ways presents the possibility of a healthy integration of a birthmother identity. In exploring the birthmother as a holistic individual, as not just damaged by relinquishment, there is the potential to study what factors, such as the provision of a doula, may contribute to an "empowered birthmother."

Doula Support

The question that remains unanswered but that this research evokes is: how does a doula affect the experiences of relinquishing women? Can doulas produce these feelings of empowerment in the face of intense stigmatization? Although this research and small sample size cannot prove a causal relationship between reports of empowerment and doula support, it is noteworthy enough to report the birthmother participants' positive experiences with their doulas.

Laura's doula was a family friend who was just beginning her career as a doula. Laura reported: "She was a lot of help as a doula, and I respected her in that professionalism aspect but not the personal aspect, which is what I wanted of her." In the "professionalism" aspect, Laura commended her doula for helping Laura have the un-medicated birth that she had desired. Laura, whose doula let her "mom take over" during the relinquishment process, had access to other forms of social support with an involved birthfather and close-knit family but still valued her doula's involvement during childbirth.

61

Elizabeth had less support from family and friends and had a doula who was also her adoption counsellor. Elizabeth benefitted from this specialized support. She relied on her doula for informational support for childbirth and the emotional support in both childbirth and relinquishment. In being estranged from her mother, Elizabeth had very little knowledge of childbirth, and since she did not acknowledge her pregnancy until her seventh month, she very quickly had to make sense of the pregnancy and childbirth process. She recalled, "I didn't understand how much was behind having a baby ... it just wasn't ever a question to me." Her doula helped her write a birth plan, which she said brought her a lot of relief as she began to consider potential complications. When Elizabeth's doula attended one of Elizabeth's prenatal appointments she

> ... brought up things that I didn't know about. About birth and pregnancy and how the whole process works and what happens when you go into having the baby and stuff. And then she brought questions up that I could ask the doctor and get informed about and what happens if something were to go wrong.... She was always there emotionally.

Elizabeth used her doula to "[talk] about anything," without judgment. Because of this ongoing support, Elizabeth felt her doula "helped a lot with the grief and everything." This level of support and its benefits make an argument for doulas attending adoptions to use a community-based doula model. Although Laura obviously benefitted from the more "professional" support from her doula in training, Elizabeth reported how much she appreciated the more engaged, expertise provided by a dual doula-adoption counsellor, saying, "I'm pretty sure I couldn't have done it without her. That sounds stupid, but she just helped me, like, know what I wanted emotionally and physically and figure out what I wanted to do, like, with the adoption and pregnancy. Just everything."

Vicki had the least support through her informal network and benefitted the most from having a doula's support. She used the same doula as Elizabeth—the doula-adoption counsellor. Vicki, like Elizabeth, had very little knowledge of pregnancy and childbirth, so she relied heavily on her doula for both informational and emotional support. Moreover, Vicki reported intense feelings of pressure to medicate during her birth: "I was like, I don't even know what that stuff does and what are the effects on the baby … they just wouldn't explain anything … the doctors don't want to explain anything. They were just like, 'Do you want this or that? What do you want? We need to know now.'" Vicki also expressed a sense of losing control since the "doctors were so rushed on everything. They wouldn't really give me a chance to think. To explain anything." She said, however, that her doula's questions and continual support empowered her to adhere to her birth plan, which she had developed with her doula. She reported a stark contrast between her doula who "already knew what I wanted" and the doctors who she felt were "persistent and trying to get it all done super quick." Vicki's fears were so allayed by her doula that she argued: "I definitely think everyone should have [a doula]. Especially if you don't know what you're getting yourself into, to have someone stand in for you and be like, 'Look, look here doctor. Here is what is going to happen. You're going to slow your roll.'" Vicki's doula was also invaluable to her for processing relinquishment. Vicki, who had relinquished only five months earlier, reported that she "definitely grieved a lot" and said "it was really hard," she confided in her doula:

[My doula] was there, still is. Just to talk to, which was great. I mean talking to [my partner] about it is different than talking to someone who deals with it. She doulas all the time for other women. She just knows the whole … she knows what it's like. It was really nice to talk to her about it. It helped a lot. It made me feel so much better.

DISCUSSION

The stories of the participants show the potential for doulas to improve birth experiences for birthmothers and ameliorate the social isolation of relinquishment. Vicki's final thoughts on her doula send a powerful message: "I couldn't imagine doing it without her." For birthmothers who are doing something that most people cannot imagine, a doula has the potential to protect against that disenfranchised grief.

✻ Doulas provide invaluable support for women as they walk into an incredibly vulnerable place. For birthmothers, childbirth is made even more vulnerable. Rather than the celebrated next step into motherhood, this is the moment of disconnect, where the reality of relinquishment is made manifest in the separation between their empty uterus and the now pink and perfect infant. For the birthmother, walking, breathing, and pushing through this space can be especially difficult. Laura fittingly phrased the odd anxiety around the separation, "She was going to be gone. I had been with her for nine months, every day. Like nonstop. So just to have her gone, like 100 percent, you know ... It was just really hard." To relinquish in a situation in which you feel that you are out of control, as many women report within biomedical births, could cause additional trauma (Devaney and Lavery 376). Research shows that doulas for "socially high risk mothers" have the potential to "increase the mother's positive feelings about labour, decrease anxiety, increase feelings of control and confidence as a mother and decrease postpartum depression" (Hans 5). Although this study did not quantitatively assess birthmother outcomes, the qualitative data support the notion that the birthmothers had positive feelings about their labour and increased feelings of control, and, although they did not need confidence as a mother, they did report confidence in relinquishing.

Doulas cannot prevent the grief associated with relinquishment, but they can support women through that loss. Social support in loss has been resoundingly proven to improve integration of loss—growth through grief (Heaney and Israel 194; Schoulte et al. 83). What if we can dare to imagine a world where the provision of doulas for birthmothers is standard practice? This is actually not an unattainable goal since most adoptive families or agencies cover the medical costs of women making a plan for adoption. This additional cost could be absorbed into family or agency contracts, and doula provision for birthmothers could become standard care. Although the emotional benefits of a doula are compelling, agencies can also realize the financial benefits of doulas from the reduction in costly interventions. The stories of the women here suggest that the simple intervention of a doula can produce profound results. Even though this strategy to improve birthmother experiences merits further examination, it is exciting to consider the ease and impact of its application by organizations and individuals seeking to support a woman making a plan of adoption.

CONCLUSION

For birthmothers, the loss that begins in birth and is compounded by the stigmatization and isolation of relinquishment provides a rich site of intervention. Research shows that an empowering birth experience may lead to empowerment in other areas such as confidence in parenting and increased rates of breastfeeding. For birthmothers, doulas may also facilitate an empowered post-re-linquishment identity.

I have mourned my loss in unexpected and exciting ways. I have, like my participants, been led to careers that seek to integrate this experience in a productive way. I have also struggled with disclosure for fear of judgment, but, ultimately, I do not feel damaged. Neither my participants nor I fit into that simple damaged birthmother model. Instead, I feel complicated by the act of relinquishing. It is complicated to love and let go, but having a doula to support a birthmother during that process may help birthmothers to take the grief, stigma and isolation and "let it go."

WORKS CITED

Aloi, Janice. "Nursing the Disenfranchised: Women Who Have Relinquished an infant for Adoption." *Journal of Psychiatric and Mental Health Nursing* 16 (2009): 27-31. Print.

Bond, M., R. Keene-Payne, and P. Lucy. "The Ideal Nurse for the Relinquishing Mother: Lessons for the Labor Room." *The American Journal of Maternal/Child Nursing* 20 (1995): 15-161. Print.

Brodzinsky, David and Susan Smith. "Post-Placement Adjustment and the Needs of Birthmothers Who Place an Infant for Adoption." *Adoption Quarterly* 17 (2014): 165-84. Print

De Simone, Michael. "Birth Mother Loss: Contributing Factors to Unresolved Grief. *Clinical Social Work Journal* 24.1 (1996): 65-76. Print.

Devaney, Susan Wuest and Sharon Farrell Lavery. "Nursing Care for the Relinquishing Mother." *Journal of Obstetric and Gynecologic Nursing* 9.60 (1980): 375-378. Print.

Ellison, Marcia A. "Authoritative Knowledge and Single Women's Unintentional Pregnancies, Abortions, Adoption and Single Motherhood: Social Stigma and Structural Violence." *Medical Anthropology Quarterly* 17.3 (2003): 322-347. Print.

Evan B. Donaldson Adoption Institute. *Benchmark Adoption Survey: Report on the Findings. Princeton Survey Research Associates.* 1997. Web. 19 Sep. 2014.

Evan, B. *Safeguarding the Rights and Well-Being of Birthparents in the AdoptionProcess.* 2007.Web. 19 Sep. 2014.

Evan, B. *National Adoption Attitudes Survey.* 2002. Web. 19 Sep. 2014.

Everson, Courtney. "Lost Cause" Mothers: Stigma, Power, and Resistance in the Performativityof Adolescent Motherhood." Presentation at American Anthropological Association 11th Meeting, San Francisco, CA. 18 Nov. 2012.

Fessler, Ann. *The Girls Who Went Away: The Hidden History of Women Who Surrendered Children for Adoption in the Decades Before Roe v. Wade.* New York: Penguin, 2007. Print.

Fisher, Allen P. "A Critique of the Portrayal of Adoption in College Textbooks and Readers on Families, 1998-2001." *Family Relations* 52.2 (2003): 154-160. Print.

Foucault, Michel. *The History of Sexuality, Vol . 1.* Harmondsworth: Penguin, 1979. Print.

Gustafson, Diana. *Unbecoming Mothers; The Social Production of Maternal Absence.* Binghamton, NY: Haworth Clinical Practice Press, 2005. Print.

Hans, Sydney. "Doula Support for Young Mothers: A Randomized Trial. Final Report."*Maternal and Child Health Bureau Research Program.* 2006. Web. 23 Sep. 2014.

Health Connect One. "The Perinatal Revolution [white paper]." Health Connect One, 2014. Web. 27 Sep. 2014.

"The Teen Parent Empowerment Program." *The Healthy Babies Project.* n.p, n.d. Web. 10 Oct.2014.

Heaney, Catherine A. and Barbara A. Israel. "Social Networks and Social Support." *Health Behavior and Health Education: Theory,*

Research and Practice. 4th ed. Eds. K. Glanz, B. K. Rimer, and K. Viswanath. Danvers, MA: Jossey-Bass, 2008. 189-210. Print.

Hodnett, E. D., S. Gates, G. J. Hofmeyr, and C. Sakala, "Continuous Support for Women duringChildbirth (Cochrane Review)." *Cochrane Database of Systematic Reviews* 3 (2007): 172. Print.

Karel, Amanda I. "Covering Adoption: General Depiction in Broadcast News." *Family Relations* 55 (2006): 487-498. Print.

Leon, Irving G. "The Role of Obstetric Caregiver in Adoption." *Primary Care Update for OB/GYNS* 6.4 (1999): 125-131. Print.

Logan, Janette. "Birth Mothers and their Mental Health: Uncharted Territory." *British Journal of Social Work* 26 (1996): 609-625. Print.

Mander, Rosemary. "The Care of the Mother Grieving a Baby Relinquished for Adoption." Aldershot, Hants: Avebury, 1995. Print.

Melosh, Barbara. *Strangers and Kin: The American Way of Adoption*. Cambridge: Harvard University Press, 2006. Print.

Oliver, Mary. *American Primitive: Poems*. Little: Brown, 1983. Print.

Pertman, Adam. *Adoption Nation: How the Adoption Revolution is Transforming America*. New York: Basic Books, 2000. Print.

Rapp, Rayna. *Testing Women, Testing the Fetus: The Social Impact of Amniocentesis ofAmerica*. New York: Routledge, 1999. Print.

Schensul, S. L., J. J. Schensul, and M. D. LeCompte. *Essential Ethnographic Methods, Vol 2: Ethnographer's Toolkit*. Walnut Creek, CA: Alta Mira, 1999. Print.

Schoulte, Joleen, Zachary Sussman, Benjamin Tallman, Munni Deb, Courtney Cornick and Elizabeth Altmaier. "Is There Growth in Grief: Measuring Posttraumatic Growth in Grief Response. *Open Journal of Medical Psychology* 1 (2012): 38-43. Print.

Ulin, Priscilla R. *Qualitative Methods: A Field Guide for Applied Research in Sexual andReproductive Health*. New York: Family Health International, 2002. Print.

Wegar, Katarina. "In Search of Bad Mothers: Social Constructions of Birth and Adoptive Motherhood." *Women's Studies International Forum* 20.31 (1997): 77-86. Print.

Winkler, Robin and Margaret van Keppel. *Relinquishing Mothers in Adoption: Their Long-Term Adjustment*. Melbourne: Institute of Family Studies, 1984. Print.

5.

"When You Go Through Something Like That with Sombebody"

Turning Points in the Relationships Between Doulas and Young Mothers

JON KORFMACHER AND MARISHA HUMPHRIES

IN HUMAN SERVICES, WHETHER ORIENTED towards health, social welfare, or emotional well-being, the helping relationship drives the service delivery. Human services are made of help-giving interactions. The service provider offers support and guidance to clients who hopefully engage with the provider and respond to the offers of assistance. This certainly applies to doulas, who offer physical comfort, reassurance, and information to mothers and their families during a time of extreme vulnerability. The success of the doula in particular depends on the development of a trusting relationship. The intimacy of childbirth demands this level of trust, and the limited time period of the relationship accentuates the need for the bond to be quickly established.

Community-based doulas typically work with families in more challenging contexts, such as low-income and low-resource neighbourhoods. They are joining with parents who often struggle with accepting help and believing that representatives from systems of care are genuinely concerned for them and their well-being (Abramson, Breedlove, and Isaacs 14; Flanagan 241). This creates both challenges and opportunities for the doula in that the mother may value having someone who can advocate and support her, even if she feels ambivalent about what a doula has to offer. The fact that doulas support the mother in the actual birth experience puts them in a unique position from other human service professionals, including most other health care providers, and provides a central event on which, it can be argued, the rest of the relationship pivots.

This makes examining the quality of the helping relationship that forms between doula and mother essential to understanding doula practice, with the birth experience as a central component of this relationship. For community-based doulas—who typically work with mothers over an extended period of time (from pregnancy through the early postpartum period)—understanding how the relationship may change over time is a priority. Before birth, the community doula's job is to directly support the mother, help her become more aware of her developing child, and anticipate welcoming the child into her life. After birth, the doula must negotiate a triadic relationship and attend to the needs of the mother and baby as well as other family members who will vary dramatically in their level of engagement.

In our previous work (Humphries and Korfmacher 26; Korfmacher 185), we delineated the key themes that emerged from in-depth interviews conducted with community-based doulas in a large metropolitan city and with the young African American mothers with whom the doulas worked. Signifiers of a positive relationship included availability, positive interactions, trust, emotional closeness, and feelings of being helped, themes that match very well with the conception of "compassionate love" (Fehr and Sprecher 39). But there were also signs of ambivalence and challenges in the relationship, including inconsistency in contact, the doula's difficulty in "reading" the mother, and doulas not accepting elements of the mother's lifestyle. In this chapter, we extend these analyses to look at how the helping relationships between the doula and the young mother changed over time, and the role that the birth experience had in this process.

Adolescence is a period marked as the preparation for adulthood (Crockett and Crouter 1). During this time, adolescents are experiencing more freedom and creating instances of choice. A significant marker during adolescence is when individuals psychologically explore who they are and how they fit it to their families, neighbourhood, and the world in general (Steinberg and Morris 91). The ability to separate from parent(s) is also a significant developmental task in the course of adolescence. During this period, relationship interests change, partly because of new and growing needs (Kirchler, Palmonari, and Pombeni 147).

Motherhood can represent one of those changing needs. The pregnant adolescent must figure out who she is as a mother during this stage of development while she also navigates multiple relationships, including those with familial and non-familial adults who have a vested interest in her both as a person and as a caregiver. The current work is particularly interested in understanding the mothers' relationship with her doula as a non-familial adult in this context of adolescent development. Research has shown that doulas who work with adolescent mothers must move beyond their roles as "doulas" if they want to facilitate positive maternal and child outcomes (Gentry et al. 36).

METHODS

Pregnant adolescent (under the age of twenty-one) African American mothers participated in a randomized intervention study examining the impact of an extended doula support model (Abramson, Breedlove, and Isaacs, 29). Of the mothers, 95 percent were considered low income and were receiving Medicaid insurance. Mothers were randomized either into a treatment condition receiving doula services (n =124) or a control condition receiving typical prenatal services at a large university clinic and hospital (n=124). A subset of mothers from the treatment condition was selected for the current qualitative study.

Participants in the current study were twelve low-income, adolescent African American mothers and their four African American female doulas. Mothers began receiving doula services towards the end of their second trimester of pregnancy, which continued until the mothers were three months postpartum. We recruited mothers who scored either high or low on a relationship security measure (Simpson 971). Eleven of the mothers were first-time mothers, a proportion similar to the overall study sample (88 percent).

The doulas ranged in age from late twenties to fifties. Three of the doulas had become mothers when they were adolescents. All doulas received four months of intensive doula training from a local community organization that developed the program model. Training focused on pregnancy, labour and childbirth, pain relief during birth, breastfeeding, responsive parenting, working with adolescent parents, and building supportive relationships. The doulas were expected to meet with the mothers weekly through home visits or during medical appointments and to maintain phone contact with mothers as needed. Doulas were expected to attend labour and delivery and to provide emotional and physical support to the mothers. They received ongoing training and supervision throughout the intervention.

Mothers were contacted a month after they initially met their doula to determine their interest in participating in this study. Mothers and doulas received monetary compensation (i.e., twenty dollars) at the end of each interview. Interviews were conducted by the second author, who is African American and who has experience conducting both research and clinical interviews. Information obtained in interviews was not shared between doulas, mothers, the doulas' supervisor, or other study administrators. Interviews lasted approximately sixty minutes (range forty-five to ninety minutes) and were audiotaped, transcribed, and checked for accuracy by the interviewer. Interview transcripts were coded by both authors.

The semi-structured interview examined the relationship between mothers and doulas. It also covered intervention services provided to the mothers as well as other beliefs and feelings that mothers and doulas had about the intervention (see Table 1). The interview was adapted from an interview used in a previous study of helping relationship development between teen mothers and paraprofessionals (Korfmacher and Marchi 22). Mothers and doulas were interviewed prenatally and two months postnatally on similar topics to maintain continuity. Through multiple readings of the interview transcripts, a code list was inductively refined. The authors additionally developed six "framing questions" that covered broad topics across each interview including the following:

•Is there a turning point in the relationship?
•Do clients and doulas agree on how they view the relationship?

Answering these framing questions after coding each transcript illuminated our agreement on the fundamental themes of the content analysis.

Table 1. *Interview Categories*

–Relationship with doula

> • *Positive signs of alliance; negative signs of alliance; areas of disagreement; role assignment of doula; time spent thinking about doula/client; change in relationship over time (second interview only)*

–Doula's relationship with child

–Relationship with family and friends

–Positive/Negative feelings toward each other

–Topics/activities/content of visits

–Perceived similarities/differences of young mother and doula

–Young mother or doula perception of program

–Staying in touch after program

–Young mother's future goals and doula support of goals

–Doula's own development

RESULTS

Three major themes emerged from the content analysis: contact, birth as a turning point, and doula flexibility. Quotes are used in this section to expound on and illustrate the themes. Pseudonyms are used in the quotes to protect the confidentiality of the participants.

Contact

Actual contact between the doula and mother was a major theme in the analysis, whether this was amount, consistency, or availability of scheduling meetings between doula and mother. This included both positive and negative dimensions of contact. As such, there were discussions regarding missed or unscheduled appointments:

> *I went to her prenatal appointment with her and we were supposed to have a visit earlier that week and she wasn't there. And so she says, "I know you are angry at me and*

you are probably going to stop working with me because this is the first time I did that." And I told her no, situations come up, we talked the situation out. She says, "Well..." It was funny the words she chose because the first thing she said was she said, "I really need you. I mean, I need to talk to you." So I told her, "You can call me whenever you need to call me." I said, "Whenever you need to call me." (Bridgette, doula)

A decrease in the amount of contact emerged as a major difference from the prenatal to the postnatal period. One doula, Ms. Donna, spoke of this issue, "Well, first of all she's definitely gotten even harder to reach, which is a normal pattern. I actually had to do a home visit at the boyfriend's house, cause that's where she spends so much of her time." The diminished amount of contact seemed, in part, to be in relation to the multiple roles and responsibilities (e.g., new mother, student, employee) the mothers were managing, so that doulas found it more challenging to contact them.

The young mothers also noted reduced contact with doulas after the birth. One doula, for instance, indicated after a difficult but successful delivery that she was expecting it to be easier to stay in touch with the client. However, it became quite difficult to establish consistent contact, and the doula noted that the contact postnatally was not as in-depth as prenatally. The young mother reported in her interview that she did not see the doula much postnatally because she was busy with the baby and school. Despite the diminished amount of contact, however, the mother also noted that she felt good about labour and delivery and was glad the doula was present for the birth.

Birth as a turning point

To what extent can the birth be considered a turning point in the relationship? In our interviews, we probed about the birth experience and the meaning that doulas and mothers placed on the event and their sharing of it with each other. Our initial thought, given the central role of the birth story in the work of the doula, was that this would be a culminating moment for the doula and young mother. Doulas and mothers certainly noted this in a number of cases. For example, one doula noted:

I still say the turning point would probably be the birth, it just seemed like it got better ... it just felt really natural. It just felt better, closer. It was more wow, we shared something, and we're sharing something now. We shared this major event in her life, and now we're sharing the new stepping stones. (Donna, doula)

For this doula, the birth facilitated a closer relationship between the doula and mother.

Often mothers discussed their initial reluctance to have the doula attend the birth. One mother mentioned concern about "this stranger massaging my back and touching my stomach and stuff like that" (Renee). Another mother noted, "I didn't want her to be in the labour room with me. I didn't care. I didn't want nobody in there except for the doctors ... because I just, people looking at me all—and then they're going to look at my facial expressions when I had her. No, but now that's like the only person I want to be there" (Veronica). The importance that this mother expressed regarding who would be looking at her face and reading her emotional state exemplifies both the intimacy of the experience and the intensity of emotions it engenders. It is a clear sign of trust and the doula's value to her that the mother comes to feel that the doula is the "only" person she wants to be with her during this event. Other mothers commented on how important and revealing the birth experience was. As one young mother, Leslie, put it, "When you go through something like that with somebody, you can't help but be emotionally attached to them. You know, because she was there. She saw the ugly side."

Despite the intensity of emotion experienced by mothers and doulas during a birth, their experience did not necessarily translate into consistent and ongoing contact after the birth of the baby. For these mothers, birth *was* a turning point in the relationship, but it was signified by a reduction of contact. Sometimes doulas were surprised to feel less connected to the mothers after the birth:

I would say that the fact that she hasn't initiated more on her own and, maybe the fact that I feel like when we are together I feel like I am doing too much talking.... It's like it's not a conversation, so she is definitely not like opening up or sharing with me. I am not exactly sure why ... maybe she needed me more [prenatally]. And so maybe that's it. Maybe she doesn't need me as much. (Donna, doula)

Interestingly, the young mother did not feel this disconnection. Even though she had less contact with her doula, she said that after the birth of the baby "she's more helpful now to me." Other mothers commented on an increased bond with their doula postnatally, as this example from Veronica's interview shows:

Q: Before you said you were kind of like sisters but you say you're even closer than you were before?
A: Yeah, because now the baby's here.
Q: And how does that make you guys closer?
A: Because she loves him just because when she met me I was pregnant and she would always talk to my stomach and now she's more closer to the baby and me.

As this quote shows, a mutual sense of joy in the baby is one way that the relationship is facilitated postnatally.

Doula Flexibility

Doulas were willing to be flexible in their work with the mothers and to meet the mothers where they were in order to deliver the best services and give the best support (Behnke and Hans 11). They would go to homes, seek out mothers at clinic visits, or meet with them in other settings. In their work, the doulas observed what they believed the mothers needed for the doula to be more effective in her work and to meet the mothers' needs. They learned that they had to adapt their role or their approach. As doula Bridgette acknowledged, "Now I've got to change again." In contrast to the feelings expressed by young mother Veronica, doula Bridgette noted with another young mother how she had to make sure that she did not pay too much attention to the newborn, even as she was tasked with promoting the initial mother-infant bond, "Wheels started turning as to how I was going to handle a home visit. How was I going to inculcate the baby in our visits but not make her feel like I'm not interested in what she needs? Or that I'm being neglectful of what she needs." It can be a delicate balance for doulas to attend to the needs of the young mothers while they incorporate the newborn into their work.

Doulas had to work to promote a sense of "mutual competence" (Bernstein 1), such as accepting that mothers may choose to bottle-feed because of their life circumstances, despite the program's heavy promotion of breastfeeding (Korfmacher 196). They acknowledged that the work also changed them and helped them recognize the value of not being too prescriptive in their approach:

> *Well, I think each experience changes you a little bit. It has changed me more. [Teresa] is one of the clients who requires more time in the program, so it taught me how to just discipline myself and give each client whatever they want. They need more time, make provisions for more time for them. She just was that one that kept me grounded to the root of the program.* (Sherry, doula)

To be successful in their work with the mothers, doulas needed to be flexible in the ways in which they interacted with the mothers and in terms of the strategies they used.

DISCUSSION

The birth experience is a focal point of the doula intervention. We know that mothers in general felt supported by their doulas during labour and delivery, both in our subset of mothers and in the overall sample from the randomized trial (Hans et al. 12). Many of the mothers, some more strongly than others, noted how helpful their doula was. As shown above, some of the mothers had mixed or negative feelings initially about their doulas joining them for the intimate nature of labour and delivery but changed their mind and came to anticipate the support that they would receive.

In most cases, however, the birth experience did not lead to consistent and ongoing contact between the mother and doula during the early newborn period, much to the doula's surprise. For many of the young mothers, the contact with their doula decreased after birth. How do we account for this? There seem to be two factors at play: i) the role of the doula after birth, including negotiating multiple relationships; and ii) the developmental identity and priorities of the adolescent.

Role Definition

The doulas in this study were expected to work with the young mothers before, during, and after birth. They were to visit mothers up to three months postpartum to promote early bonding and help in the transition to motherhood. Although the community-based doula model proposes this extended role for the doula, much of the initial doula training focused on the support for the birth process. Doulas themselves saw this as their primary function and a way to distinguish their role from conventional home visitors. One implication of this focus is that doulas found it more challenging to conceptualize the best way to provide support during the newborn period. From providing emotional support and physical comfort to the mother to negotiating the relationship between the new parent and the child, as well as providing caregiving advice and guidance—the doulas' role was less defined and also altered. Closing one chapter of the mother's journey with the close and emotionally-laden birth experience may have made it more difficult for the doula and mother to move on together to the next chapter of emerging parenthood, where the mother-child dyad becomes the central relationship.

To a greater extent after birth, doulas also had to deal with extended members of the mother's family, including the young mother's own mother. This often involved working through conflicting childcare advice, such as infant feeding (see Korfmacher 198). Another issue that emerged postpartum was deciding when it was appropriate for the doula to visit the young mother. The doula training model strongly encourages frequent contact with the mother during the early perinatal period as a unique window of opportunity, as this is the time that key decisions around breastfeeding and other early bonding experience are made (Abramson, Breedlove, and Isaacs 35). Doulas, however, were ambivalent about these meetings because they felt that they were potentially intruding on a time that should be reserved for immediate family. Their desire to be respectful of family priorities came at the cost of delayed and inconsistent contact with the family during a key transition point of the service. This likely also exacerbated the doulas' role confusion with the young mothers postnatally.

Adolescent Development

Adolescents begin to spend less time with their parents and more time with friends, romantic partners, or even alone. This shift in the use of personal time may affect the amount of time that the adolescent mothers want (or have) to spend with their doulas. The young mothers typically conceptualized their relationships with their doulas in personal terms (e.g., a friend or family member), but they did not view their doula as a same-age peer. Even though the relationship had personal qualities similar to that of a peer, the doulas worked hard to maintain a helper role, which put them at some level of authority. This may help to explain reduced availability of the adolescent mother for visits with the doula after birth, despite feeling emotionally close to the doula.

Another developmental issue to consider is the adolescent's relationship with a non-familial adult. Is it developmentally appropriate to expect that an adolescent mother would have a mutually collaborative relationship with her doula in the same way that an adult mother would? Conceptions of doula-adolescent mother relationships may need to be adjusted to reflect the realities of adolescent development. The experiences reported by the mothers and doulas during labour and delivery demonstrated the emotional closeness of the relationship between them. However, this emotional closeness did not translate into increased contact as we expected. In our previous paper (Humphries and Korfmacher 29) we noted this dichotomy between reduced contact yet continued feelings of connection as a sign of "ambivalence" in the relationship, in that these feelings of warmth and trust were not enough to lead to a solid and consistent partnership. However, if one views the relationship through a developmental lens, this distinction between the amount of contact and feelings of closeness may not be so surprising, as the expected positive association between closeness and contact may simply not be reflective of an adolescent relationship.

Despite feeling emotionally close to their doula after the birth, mothers often want to return to the life of a "teenager." Several mothers noted that not only were they adjusting to the demands of being a mother but they were also returning to school, returning to or entering the work force, having romantic relationships, and maintaining their high school social lives. As a result, the mothers were very busy after the birth, leading to less time to meet with their doulas. Barlow and colleagues (203) found in their research with young, vulnerable mothers that mothers were less likely to engage in supportive programs when they felt overburdened by other life circumstances. Similarly, a qualitative examination of the Nurse Family Partnership home visiting program in Memphis found that young African American mothers served by the program typically had many family and filial obligations during the day. Their commitments were so much that nurses often struggled to keep track of and make contact with their clients, despite the mother's professed interest in remaining in the program (Kitzman, Cole, Yoos, and Olds 103).

CONCLUSION

The relationship between a doula and mother serves as a critical element in the effectiveness of a doula intervention, but this relationship can be more complicated with adolescent mothers. The closeness of the relationship and the emotional intensity of the birth experience did not translate into consistent contact between the doula and the young mother during the final three months of the program. Doulas themselves need to be mindful about their changing role with the family and how this will impact the time that they will spend with the new mother. Future research should explore young mothers' expectations and their conceptions of the roles of doulas and other helping professions to maximize the effectiveness of service delivery during this unique window of opportunity in the life of a young family.

WORKS CITED

Abramson, Rachel, Ginger Breedlove, and Beth Isaacs. *The Community Based Doula: Supporting Families Before, During, and After Childbirth*. Washington, DC: ZERO TO THREE Press, 2006. Print.

Barlow, Jane, Sue Kirkpatrick, Sarah Stewart-Brown, and Hilton Davis. "Hard-to-Reach or Out-of-Reach? Reasons Why Women Refuse to Take Part in Early Interventions." *Children & Society* 19.3 (2005): 199-210. Print.

Behnke, Erin and Sydney Hans. "Becoming a Doula." *ZERO TO THREE* 23.2 (2002): 9-13. Print

Bernstein, Victor. "Strengthening Families through Strengthening Relationships: Supporting the Parent-Child Relationship through Home Visiting." *IMPrint: Newsletter of the Infant Mental Health Promotion Project 35* (2002-2003): 1-5. Print.

Crockett, Lisa J. and Ann C. Crouter. "Pathways through Adolescence: An Overview." *Pathways through Adolescence: Individual Development in Relation to Social Contexts*. Eds. Lisa J. Crockett and Ann C. Crouter. Mahwah, NJ: Lawrence Erlbaum Associates, Publishers, 1995. 1-12. Print.

Fehr, Beverly and Susan Sprecher. "Compassionate Love: Conceptual, Measurement, and Relational Issues." *The Science of Compassionate Love: Theory, Research, and Applications*. Eds. Beverley Fehr, Susan Sprecher, and Lynn G. Underwood. San Francisco: Wiley-Blackwell, 2008. 27–52. Print.

Flanagan, Patricia. "Teen Mothers: Countering the Myths of Dysfunction and Developmental Disruption." *Mothering Against the Odds: Diverse Voices of Contemporary Mothers*. Eds. Cynthia Garcia-Coll, J. L. Surrey, and K. Weingarten. New York: Guilford Press, 1998. 238–254. Print.

Gentry, Quinn M., Kim M. Nolte, Ainka Gonzalez, Magan Person, and Symeon Ivey. "'Going Beyond the Call of Doula': A Grounded Theory Analysis of the Diverse Roles Community-Based Doulas Play in the Lives of Pregnant and Parenting Adolescent Mothers." *The Journal of Perinatal Education* 19.4 (2010): 24-40. Print.

Hans, Sydney, Linda Henson, Jon Korfmacher, Luara Walton, Kate Pickett, and John Lantos. "Doula Prenatal and Birth Support for

Young Socially Vulnerable Mothers: A Randomized Controlled Trial." Manuscript in preparation. University of Chicago, 2015. Print.

Humphries, Marisha L. and Jon Korfmacher. "The Good, the Bad, and the Ambivalent: Quality of Alliance in a Support Program for Young Mothers." *Infant Mental Health Journal* 33.1 (2012): 22-33. Print.

Kirchler, Erich, Augusto Palmonari, and Maria L Pombeni. "Developmental Tasks and Adolescents' Relationships with their Peers and their Family." *Adolescence and Its Social Worlds*. Eds. Sandy Jackson and Hector Rodriguez-Tome. Est Sussex, UK: Lawrence Erlbaum Associates, 1993. 145-168. Print

Kitzman, Harriet., Robert Cole, Lorrie Yoos, and David Olds. "Challenges Experienced by Home Visitors: A Qualitative Study of Program Implementation". *Journal of Community Psychology,* 25.1 (1997): 95–109. Print.

Korfmacher, Jon. "Supporting Parents Around Feeding and Eating in Early Childhood." *Eating Behaviors of the Young Child: Prenatal and Postnatal Influences on Healthy Eating*. Eds. Leanne Birch and William Dietz. Elk Grove Village, IL: American Academy of Pediatrics, 2007: 185-203. Print.

Korfmacher, Jon, and Isabela Marchi. "The Helping Relationship in a Paraprofessional Teen Parenting Program." *ZERO TO THREE* 23.2 (2002): 21-26. Print.

Simpson, Jeffry A. "Influence of Attachment Styles on Romantic Relationships. *Journal of Personality and Social Psychology* 59 (1990): 971–980. Print.

Steinberg, Laurence and Amanda Sheffield Morris. "Adolescent Development." *Annual Review of Psychology* 52 (2001): 83-110. Print.

6.
Doulas as Facilitators
of Transformation and Grief

AMY L. GILLILAND

Grief is a process towards attaining a new identity, rather than a state. —Colin Murray Parkes

MANY OF US ARE FAMILIAR WITH the role of the doula as emotional and physical support during labour. Yet it is important to also recognize the role that doulas play during life changes and shifting relationships. Life changes always involve loss and grief over what has shifted. It is in this tender territory of loss where doulas in this study revealed their strength as facilitators of transformation. This chapter examines the processes of grief, transformation, and the function of the doula as a "wise witness" and "trusted guide." Research shows that doulas are most effective when they are not friends or family members and a prenatal relationship exists (Hodnett). Doula skills are relationship based. Many emotional support strategies employed by doulas are sophisticated and are employed by skilled counsellors as well. (Gilliland "Emotional Support Strategies"). Doulas are engaged by mothers and their intimate family to be guides through the process of pregnancy and birth. While mothers are initiated into their maternal responsibilities by the health care system, fathers may feel that they have no place in the societal rituals of pregnancy (Shibli-Kometiani; Finnbogadottir). The doula fills that gap, treating clients as a pregnant couple if that is their desire. She morphs her services to meet their presenting needs.

The mothers in my study who had their choice of doulas selected her[1] because they felt safe on an intuitive level. Most of the mothers who met their doula once labour had started said they felt a sense of connection and ease with her. Because of the massive changes brought by pregnancy and the intensity of labour, women and men's fears and needs for comfort are magnified. The doula is trusted; the person who never leaves, the one who holds the barf bag, and dries the tears. It is only natural that she is looked to for comfort when deeper issues surface. In my research uncovering the mechanism for doula effectiveness (Gilliland "Effective Labor"), there were several mothers and doulas who spoke in their interviews about grief and transformation. Mothers grieved for their lost former life, for who they thought they would be in labour, and for the birth they didn't achieve. Sometimes the loss was literal for the baby or husband who had died during the pregnancy. In all situations, the doula was trusted to provide guidance and show them the way to their new life and integrate their experience.

METHODS

From 2002 to 2010, I interviewed twenty-nine independent practice doulas, fourteen hospital-based or program doulas, twenty-two mother-father pairs, ten mothers and one father about their experiences with birth doula labour support. Doula participants were from from ten different states in the U.S. and two Canadian provinces and practised in large and small cities, and in rural areas. Participants came from various economic classes, religious faiths, and ranged in age from twenty-eight to sixty. Doulas needed to be eighteen years or older, to speak English fluently, to have attended at least twenty-five births, and to not have used clinical obstetrical or midwifery skills in any capacity. The parents were from four different states in the U.S. and lived in cities or rural areas. They ranged from twenty-five to thirty-eight years old. Participants did not need to be married; however, a close family member needed to be present for the entire labour and birth, which was usually the father, in addition to the doula. The mother's doula attended continuously from the beginning of active labour until several hours after the baby was born. Caesarean deliveries were included in the study as they account for approximately 33 percent of all U.S. births (Martin et al.). None of the participating mothers received labour support from doulas who participated in this study. Detailed description of recruitment processes, data analysis, and sample description has been published elsewhere (Gilliland "Effective Labor").

Snowball sampling was used for recruitment of participants. Open sampling in a grounded theory study requires only that interviewees be relevant to the research question (Strauss and Corbin). After approval was received from the University of Wisconsin-Madison Internal Review Board, recruitment efforts began via several doula email networks. Interviews were audiotaped and conducted in hotel rooms or living rooms. Analysis of the data was conducted through grounded theory methods using the itemized procedures of Strauss and Corbin. This method is especially suited for examining human interaction and examining the functions and processes being described by participants. This chapter uncovers themes on identity, birth, and loss through an examination of the processes of transformation, grief, and the function of the doula as a wise witness and trusted guide.

"WHO AM I NOW?"

Birth is transforming, for to become a mother, the maiden in her must die. She will remember that self but never again be that self. As Doula Alison[2] pointed out:

> [Mothers] always talk about sleep by saying, "I can't wait for it to get back to normal." I say, "You will never sleep the same way again a day in your life. I don't care if your baby is three months old or thirty-five, you will not sleep the same way again. I don't care if that child's in the house or not. You will go to bed every night wondering how that child is wherever they are in the world."

Repeatedly, doulas told how they reassured mothers and fathers that these feelings of loss and uncertainty were normal. Sometimes this happens during labour, as Camille, a birth doula who had attended seventy-five births recalled:

The baby was starting to crown and she said, "Oh, I'm so afraid." I was whispering to her, "You know what? Only the part of you who's not a mom is going to die. The rest, you're not going to die." And she was like, "Oh! Okay." You know? Sometimes it is that simple of somebody telling you, "I recognize that you have this fear and it's a pretty normal fear to have."

Surrendering to the process of becoming a new version of your self can be daunting. The normal is what is happening now in this moment. It will never be again as it is now, and it will change again once the baby is born. Alison told this story to illustrate this point:

She was kind of weepy, and that's when it hit me, she's not done being a CNN producer yet. And she can't be a CNN producer and have this baby ... so I said to her, "What's it like having this come three weeks before?" She's like, "I just wasn't ready. I thought I was going to have three weeks to read all those books and to do this and to do that." ...So you're sad that you're leaving that, and you're leaving it before you were emotionally ready to leave it, because you hadn't gone through that three-week grieving process that you thought you were going to get before your baby was actually due? And she was like, "Yeah." And she started to really tear up and everything, and I said, "That's okay. Just be sad for that."

Part of the role of trusted guide is normalizing the fears and doubt of the labour process as Alison did. Mothers also talked about this shift in identity. Their interviews revealed their process of making meaning of their experience to define who they were now. First time mother Gail compared herself to her sister:

My sister, who's eighteen months younger than me, has two kids and she had a fifty-hour labour, at home with a tub and back labour. And so I consistently still think, well, why couldn't I go fifty hours? I only made twenty-eight hours [before any pain medication] ... I don't know if that

means that I had more pain or less management of the pain
or was more of a wuss, or what. I don't know what to
do with that fact. I'm still really wrestling with that fact.

Gail acknowledged her doula's efforts to explain that the labour
was extraordinarily difficult. She felt her feelings were reflected and
validated. But in the end, the responsibility of creating a meaning
that works for Gail is her own. Similarly, another mother, Georgia,
struggled with comparing herself to others, including her sister,
mother-in-law, and friends. She was upset with herself for screaming and crying during her un-medicated three-hour active labour.
Georgia recalled: "I grieve about weird things ... I felt like a failure
for a week that I was in so much pain that I was screaming. And
[his mother] is so exaggerating, everything is so painful to her and
she's always screaming and crying. So if she didn't scream during
her birth, then I must be like the biggest wimp ever." Eventually
Georgia went on to conclude, "I guess I'm really hard on myself
because all of my friends have done everything totally traditionally,
I don't know if any of this haunts them ... I think in time I'm going
to be totally fine with it."

As Georgia and Gail try to make sense of their births, their emphasis is on answering the questions: Who am I? What does my
birth say about me? And how do I define myself now? They both
described their doula's communication as being reflective of their
own process, which can be seen as guiding them to their new selves.

"RESOLVING THE BIRTH"

Grieving for the birth experience one wanted goes beyond a birth
not meeting a mother's expectations. Healing from and resolution
of the birth experience means deeply feeling the emotions that arise
and coming to terms with the birth's personal symbolic meaning
in one's life. It often means going through each of the five stages
of grief as defined by Kubler-Ross (2005). In the first stage, denial
or shock, the person may not realize the depth of the experience's
meaning. They may understate what happened or even seem to
not realize what is going on. Eventually denial gives way to anger
and wondering how things might have been different. Stating "if

only" is the hallmark of the bargaining part of the process. With sadness comes the realization that what happened is awful and that life has irrevocably changed. With time, acceptance becomes the norm—the experience and its meaning are integrated into our new identities. While these stages are overlapping and somewhat sequential, they are experienced more like a pendulum. A person can move from anger to sadness and then to acceptance and back to bargaining and then even to denial. Eventually, though, acceptance comes to rule. Gail was grieving for the birth she wanted but didn't have. In this passage, the five stages defined by Kubler-Ross can be heard in Gail's story:

> *At that point I said I wanted an epidural. There was fi-*
> *nally a point where I couldn't manage any more. And I'm*
> *just very sad about that. I feel really sad, and a little mad*
> *because I wonder, What if we had practiced more, what*
> *if I had tried more things? What if I had been at home,*
> *where I didn't have the option? What difference would*
> *that have made? Or what if I didn't feel like I had to go*
> *to the hospital when my water broke? What if I'd felt*
> *like I didn't have to even induce myself, do the natural*
> *inductions, would my labour have been different ... would*
> *I have managed better at home with a lot of this? So I'm*
> *very regretful. I guess the point on the other side, I feel*
> *like I had, for me, unbearable pain, and so I was happy*
> *that there was an epidural that could help me.... So I think*
> *that my coming to terms is not going to be through saying*
> *the support should have been this or that, it's going to be*
> *more a broader acceptance of what birth is and can be, and*
> *allowing my birth to be what it was and not second-guess*
> *myself quite as much. I'm very judgmental about myself*
> *and I need to keep letting that go.*

Here we hear Gail's voice as she processes her experience. She grieves the birth, but there is also the thread of acceptance and transformation present. As Gail described the postpartum meetings with her doula, Gail acknowledged her own reluctance to discuss what happened. Instead, she focused on the baby and breastfeeding.

Yet she expressed that her doula was who she needed to talk with, and she anticipated her kindness and compassion.

In narratives from both mothers and doulas, doulas were seen as trusted guides and wise witnesses who understood the emotions of grief and did not shy away from their intensity. Doula Angela told this story:

> *She was really trying so hard to have a vaginal birth, but it just didn't work. And she said she was okay with it, but I could see that she wasn't. I made a trek out to see her, and I brought her a journal and told her that, "If you can't tell me that story and you can't tell anyone else, please write it down and get it out." Because I think she just was keeping it inside, she'd replay it over and over and over in her head. I said, "When you write it down, share it with someone. I will come back...."*

In her doula role as a wise witness, Angela backed up the mother's perceptions of her birth rather than invalidating them by sharing her own. She attempted to guide her client through this process at the clients' timing, not her own. Grief is not reconciled easily or quickly. It takes time. In all of these instances the mothers had not yet concluded their relationship with their doulas. They knew there was more support available to them. In this way, the doula served as a wise witness or someone who understood what happened at their birth and whose role was to be present during their healing process.

"LOSS"

The theme of loss also emerged as doulas spoke of their role at a fetal demise or when the husband was unable to be present or had died during the pregnancy. Sometimes, the doula needed to help process the mother's grief during the labour. When mothers had a few days between the baby's death and labour, they often moved past the denial stage. Tierney was a doula and hospital social worker at several dozen fetal demise labours and births. She said that the labour support tasks were the same—helping women to get the information they needed to make decisions, offering emotional support and providing coping measures. The doulas in the study who attended a labour where the baby was known to already be dead stated that mothers sometimes had irrational thoughts, mood swings and emotional releases. The doulas said their role was to accept her and use the same emotional support skills, to serve as a trusted guide in this unexpected territory. What is different, which is apparent in Delia's account below, is that the doula also had emotional responses. However, she realized that even though the event affected her emotionally, it was not centred on her. In all three stories shared by doulas in this section, doulas dealt with their own emotions after leaving the families.

Doula Delia tells about the first fetal demise she attended. Her story demonstrates the emotional support skills of an experienced doula: encouraging, explaining, accepting, reinforcing, and re-framing (Gilliland "Effective Labor"). She also advocated for the mother and connected her to her care team:

> She called me and said, "I haven't felt the baby move and we're on the way to the hospital. What do you think?" I said, "Sweetie, I don't know. But you're being a good parent and you're on your way to the hospital...." Time goes on and on and I'm getting to be a wreck. Get a phone call from the dad, "There's no heartbeat and would you please come?" All the family is there. Dad walks out of the OR and the baby was gone. They tried to resuscitate and no chance. It was cord strangulation and must have happened overnight. Baby was moving fine the day before and she went to bed and she lost her. And he just came out, "Oh my God, what are we going to do?" Just weeping, all the family around weeping. And you're numb. And so you start lending support. Of just holding and loving and, "This is difficult." And there are no words to say. But I did the best that I knew to do and that was to call the woman that runs the bereavement program. The nursing staff said, "Oh, she's not on call today." I said, "Will you page her? Just page her. I don't care." And they did ... it turns out she supported the [mom's twin] sister who had

lost a baby. So the connection was there.

I went into recovery and Mom is looking at me, "What did I do? What did I do?" They didn't give her a reason as to why the baby was gone. The nurse was whispering under the breath, "There's nothing she could do, the baby was gone." I said, "Tell her, give her the truth right now. It's what she needs." So [the nurse] looked at me and I said, "Go over and tell her right now," and she did ... I checked on all the family—"Do you need food? Do you need something to drink? Are there any phone calls I can make for you?" Then they have the procedure of bathing the baby, dressing the baby and having mom see the baby, and family members hold the baby. I was allowed to do that. So I got to bathe this precious little thing and dress her and make sure her hair was combed, and put booties on her. I put a bow in her hair and wrapped her up beautifully and then presented her to her parents. It was very difficult. Personally for me it brought up a lot of memories. I had a sister-in-law who was tragically killed at nine months pregnant with my niece twenty years ago. And I was the first person who went to hold my niece ... (pauses). I helped work out funeral arrangements, stayed on call for this family, took the husband to the funeral home, just whatever they needed I was there for the family. [I put my] feelings aside but when I did get home, (sighs heavily) ... there was my husband, just holding me and sobbing. I'd lost a baby. It was awful.

In Delia's moving story, we are able to envision the strategies that she employed in service of her clients. She gives excellent examples of often used skills and techniques employed in a slightly different way. She was still functioning as a guide even though the context was new to her. It is important to note that Delia never stopped doula-ing: the focus remained on the family members and supporting them. It was not about her own experience or grief but about theirs. Several doulas in the study said that they had taken courses at the hospital to help prepare the babies' bodies for the parents. They knew how to do the memory box materials and how to reassure and explain to parents what to expect.

Similarly, another experienced doula, Lydia, explained what she did when the baby died postpartum in the hospital:

> *They were going to release her Monday afternoon and this*
> *happened Monday morning. She rolled over on her baby*
> *and suffocated it. Her husband called me and said, "Please*
> *come to the hospital. They took the baby out of the room,*
> *she's not breathing." And I didn't even know at that point*
> *what had happened. So I went to the hospital. I spent the*
> *entire day Monday at the hospital with her. Then Monday*
> *evening, he asked me to go to their apartment. Because it*
> *was obvious at that point that the baby wasn't going to*
> *make it. And I went to her apartment and I took all the*
> *baby stuff out. The crib, you know, everything. Everything*
> *out. It's only been a week and half ago that that stuff got*
> *moved out of my house. [Four months later] ... Every time*
> *I walked through my front door, I saw it. It was just one*
> *more reminder.*

It is clear from both Lydia's and Delia's stories that doulas also grieve for these lost babies and hurting parents. Doula work is heart work that cannot be accomplished effectively without giving of oneself. It requires authentic connection between people, especially when the mother is in a transformative space.

In this last passage, doula Shenise described her commitment to a mother whose husband was killed in the twin towers on 9/11. Her role as a wise witness permeates her time with this family. Even though she had attended over five hundred mothers in labour, Shenise still felt vulnerable and had her own doubts and uncertainties. In this detailed excerpt, from their first meeting through postpartum, the themes of transformation, loss, and grief for both the mother and the doula are apparent:

> *I love doing prenatal visits, and I drive to them without*
> *a thought. And that day that I was going to do that first*
> *visit, it was not a thoughtless travel. There was a lot of*
> *anxiety. What do I say? What do I do? How do I be? How*

do I acknowledge this incredible tragedy? And so I drove there and I actually parked down the block. Cause I knew I just needed to be ... So when I felt okay, I pulled in the driveway and got out. She met me at the door and I knew I just had to say "I'm so sorry." Once I said that, she just burst into tears. I didn't know her, but I immediately went to touch her. She hugged me and we kind of embraced for five minutes of just tears.

Then when she was ready, she showed me pictures of him. I was able to really learn about him and what their marriage had been. And about September 11th. He was an officer on his way up. He had called from the forty-third floor and was on his way up when the tower went down. She was really able to just share a lot of intimate details about that—which is not your typical doula meeting. We weren't talking about birth. We were talking about death, and we were talking about relationships. After we had really explored that, I was able to ask her how was she feeling about the pregnancy. And move into the birth. This was her third baby. She had two Caesarean sections and was planning a third. Her baby was due a week after her husband's birthday. At a prenatal visit that he was at, he had joked, "Why don't we just schedule it for my birthday?" So when she went to the physician after September 11th, the doctor said "Why don't we schedule it for his birthday, he would have liked that." On that day we talked a lot about her preferences for a Caesarean. What were her choices? She was not aware that she could have her baby after the birth. All her babies had been whisked off to the nursery. And she didn't know about the breast crawl. She had breastfed all her children but was unaware that there could be a different intimacy in the first hour....

She went into labour before the birth date would have come, and I met her at the hospital.... And it was wonderful because her two girlfriends were there. We made this circle of women around her. She was in very early labour, so she wasn't uncomfortable yet. So they were getting ready to do the Caesarean and they had to wait because she had had lunch. We had moments of incredible tears. Of really talking about her husband not being there and the baby's father not being present. And then this breeze would come through. And we would lighten, and we would talk about the baby, or we would talk about some other subject. There would be laughter in the room. And if you walked in, you would've just thought we were a group of women laughing. Her sister-in-law went into the OR with her. They only allowed one person. But they allowed her friends and me to be waiting in recovery.

They had never ever allowed a baby in the hospital to go into recovery, always the baby went right into the nursery. This was a big exception. People gathered around, and the baby was immediately skin-to-skin on her, and it was an incredible moment. She looked at the baby, and she looked at us, and she said, "She has her father's eyes. It's so good to see his eyes again." I could feel both the joy and the depths of sorrow in it simultaneously. Some fellow officers and friends gathered and they were in the hallway, very emotional. We kept all the men out until the baby did the breast crawl. Her friend filmed it, and she was so amazed. Nurses came in. A physician came in. They said, "I've never ever seen a baby do this." The mother was so in awe that her baby had this ability and that she never separated from her baby. She said, "Thank you so much, this was such a wonderful gift of a doula." To be able to facilitate a really special beginning at a time that she so much needed to have that new beginning—it made me feel really good to be able to be there for that, even though it was so hard to share the depths of grief and the joy and heights of birth simultaneously. I'd never felt it to the extreme, even when I've been at births where there's a loss. So to have loss, death, and life simultaneously was really incredible.

Birth can be a simple transition from maiden to mother. It can be a journey fraught with fear, extraordinary pain, and uplifting joy. Doula, mother, and parent narratives revealed that doulas are seen as trusted guides and wise witnesses. In their trusted guide role, doulas ushered people through the intensity of an event by meeting their needs in the moment. They were calm in the face of strong emotion and allowed the experiences to unfold. Doulas made suggestions and asked leading questions, knowing that connecting the mother to her own wisdom was important. Besides being a knowledgeable guide, these narratives revealed the doula as a wise witness. They were present to what was happening but wise enough to offer support and not advice. Mothers and fathers felt connected to someone who understood what they were going through. Doulas did not rush them or offer their own points of view invalidating those of the parents. This made the processes of transformation and integration easier whether it was resolving what happened at their birth, integrating a change in identity, or coping with the loss of a baby or partner.

To participate in this intimate labour, doulas needed to be emotionally vulnerable. As witnesses, they risked being hurt and having powerful memories stored in their brains for years. It was not only the parents who were grieving and transformed but also the doulas. Many of the doulas in this study stated that grief and transformation of self are part of being a doula—they see themselves as the caring heart of the birth team. The doula's caring came without the strings of a personal agenda or having personal needs to be met. The doula was focused on meeting the mother's and her partner's needs. Because of this, she was free to guide transformation and navigate the terrain of grief for each mother and her family.

ENDNOTES

[1]Doulas in this study identified as cisgendered women, although there are male and transgender doulas.
[2]All names are pseudonyms.

WORKS CITED

Finnbogadottir, H., E. C. Svalenius, and E. K. Persson. "Expectant

First-Time Fathers' Experiences of Pregnancy." *Midwifery* 19.2 (2003): 96-105. Print.

Gilliland, Amy .L." After Praise and Encouragement: Emotional Support Strategies Used by Birth Doulas in the USA and Canada. *Midwifery* 27.4 (2011): 525-531. Print.

Gilliland, Amy L. *A Grounded Theory Study of Effective Labor Support by Doulas.* Diss.University of Wisconsin-Madison, 2010. Print.

Hodnett, Ellen, S. Gates, G. J. Hofmeyr and C. Sakala. "Continuous Support for Women During Childbirth." *Cochrane Database of Systematic Reviews* 7 (2013): n. pag. Web. 16 Nov. 2015.

Kubler-Ross, Elizabeth, *On Grief and Grieving: Finding the Meaning of Grief Through the Five Stages of Loss.* New York: Simon & Schuster Ltd, 2005. Print.

Martin, J.A., E. Brady, B. E. Hamilton, M. J. Osterman, S. Curtin, and T. Mathews. "Births: Final Data for 2012. National Vital Statistics Reports." *National Center for Health Statistics* 62.9 (2013): n. pag. Web. 16 Nov. 2015.

Shibli-Kometiani, M. and A. M. Brown. "Fathers' Experiences Accompanying Labour and Birth." *British Journal of Midwifery* 20.5 (2012): 339-344. Print.

Strauss, Anselm and Juliet Corbin. "Grounded Theory Methodology." *Strategies of Qualitative Inquiry.* Eds. N. Denzin and Y. Lincoln.Thousand Oaks, CA: Sage Publication, 1998. 158-183. Print.

II.
Doulas and Their Community

7.
Learning to Walk in Water

Invoking Yemanja on the Doula Path

MARIA E. HAMILTON ABEGUNDE

I AM AN *EGUNGUN* (ANCESTRAL) PRIEST and a devotee of the
Yoruba *orisa* (energy/deity) Osun.[1] I take care of the ancestors,
those yet to be born, and the living. As a devotee of Osun,
it also means that I work from a place of love and compassion,
creating rituals and ritual spaces that empower both. As a Carib-
bean-American woman, my healing work has focused on learning
about and improving the lives of other beings, especially the lives
of Black people throughout the world. A good part of what I do
involves teaching children, yet I have never given birth to my own.
Five years ago, if you had asked me to list my primary obligations,
I would have listed caring for the ancestors, the dead, as one of
the highest. It took moving to Indiana for me to be initiated fully
into my path as a daughter of Osun, the alpha and the breath of
life called into being.

How have I found myself in Bloomington, Indiana, a small
city with only a 4.6 percent (*American FactFinder*) Black or African-American population (fewer than four thousand people),
many of whom remain invisible outside of the handful of friends
that I have. How have I found myself doing something that I never
dreamed of doing? How can I take my first steps as a doula and
live in a community who is suspicious of my religion and spiritual
practice, and who do not always consider my history and Black-
ness beautiful?

For a year now, I have been walking in water at high tide. If
you have ever done this, especially in the ocean, you know how
difficult it is. Sand, shells, rocks, small fish, and seaweed slow you

down; you become distracted by the smell of salt, the sight of other bathers, the sky reflected in the water. The current constantly folds across your legs and torso like a heavy canvas. Several times in your journey from the beach to the edge of nowhere, you must stop either from exhaustion or a sudden desire to know how long you can remain still or tread water against the pushing of the waves. Or sometimes you stop because you know that one more step will plunge you up to your nose in water. Yet experience has taught me that I can't stand still for long, and I can't move very far without yearning for the warm water to cover me, without wanting to surrender to my need to be held up effortlessly and unconditionally, without thinking *this is what it means to be inside a loving mother's womb*. It is not the heaviness of my body or my inability to swim well that will sink me. Fear and a belief that I am alone will do this. It is my knowledge that the *orisa* Yemanja rocks me in the palm of her hand that keeps me afloat.

Yemanja: Mother of the Fishes. Mother of the Ocean, Protector of Women, Children, Queer Communities, and Sailors. The Mother Who Has Room for All of Humanity, She Who feeds Us from the Infinite Bounty of the Sea. She is so powerful and fluid that, like water, She cannot be contained, is not predictable, and Her form cannot be restricted. Choosing the doula path has meant choosing Yemanja and learning about what it means to be a mother, something I will not biologically experience. Moving to Indiana has also forced me to accept my connection to Yemanja, one that meant I had to remember who I am.

I grew up on the ocean in a place called La Taste in St. Patrick parish, on the island of Grenada. My childhood pictures show me sitting with my back to the water or appearing afraid to step into it. In the photos, I am never in the water, even when my own mother tries to guide me gently to it. Yet I have clear memories of being comforted by the waves against my body and holding my breath while I dived under to see what was at the bottom. It would not be until decades later when I was visiting Brazil, home to the largest and most famous Yemanja festival in the Americas, that I would ask: What does Yemanja have to do with me?

Everything about Yemanja is full and cyclical, Black, and African. She is one of the Great spiritual Mothers of the Yoruba people who survived the Middle Passage, the horrific sea voyage that carried millions of Africans from Africa to the Americas and Caribbean. When not represented as a double-tailed mermaid, Yemanja is depicted as a dark-skinned Black woman with large breasts and big hips. The bounty of the sea surrounds her as she breastfeeds a child. Contemporary images and practices related to Yemanja vary. In Brazil, she can appear as a dark-skinned woman or as a woman with long flowing hair, pure white skin, and blue eyes.[22] How Yemanja becomes the female *orisa* represented as dark skinned can be traced to several evolutions in history and cultural practices. For example, in nineteenth-century Cuba, as in many countries where Africans and their descendants were enslaved, motherhood and slavery for Black women were inextricably linked. Elizabeth Perez writes that in Cuba "motherhood was ... shaped by racial discourses ... the economy of slavery..." and that Yemanja came to be associated with the Virgin of Regla, "the only Marion icon in Cuba considered to be of direct African descent" (Perez 9-10).

During slavery, Afro-Cuban women may have recognized in the dark-skinned Virgin's face their own faces, in her full body their own bodies, and in her nursing of the baby Jesus their own sub-jugation and lower hierarchal placement by males. By associating the Virgin with Yemanja, it was also possible for the women to find strength in both figures as queens, creators of "everlasting life," protectors, and nourishers of children without abandoning their African heritage (Perez 13-20). This association is one of the many ways that the Yoruba subsumed their own religion into that of their colonizers' as an act of resistance against domination that eventually ensured the religion's survival into the twenty-first century and its practice by devotees of different races and cultures (Jones 325-326). Like water, she has the ability to move and change all in her path, as gently as a river or as forceful as a tsunami, *and* she has the power to heal. Notwithstanding these characteristics and her African birth and heritage, it is Yemanja's love and nur-ture of difference, her strength to protect those who are more at risk, and her commitment to guide her devotees through difficult times, that makes her accessible, like the Virgin Mary, to many people worldwide. Like the Virgin, Yemanja turns no one away and welcomes everyone under her skirts.

While swimming and sailing the Atlantic Ocean, I have learned many lessons from Yemanja, lessons that now translate to my new role as a doula: before entering, offer the ocean a small gift or prayer; enter with respect; be mindful always; listen for the change in the tide; allow her to guide me to the safe places; the first wave in a set hits the hardest; the subsequent waves in the set can be timed; the hand behind my back will support me; do not turn away from the water for long; cry when necessary; attend to the invisible and the inaudible; pay attention.

I carry these lessons with me from the beach to the birthing room. When I enter the latter, I am mindful that I have entered an external womb that contains the inner womb of the mother preparing to give birth. I have entered, therefore, a level of the cosmos and consciousness that exists between dimensions. Before I enter the room, I ready (and steady) myself by agreeing to be present but invisible: this moment, no matter how long, is not my moment.

As a doula, I have had to deepen my healing skills to learn how in nine months one body will become a multiple. At my first meeting with a mother-to-be, the most powerful thing I can do is what Yemanja has always done for me: listen. The next powerful thing I can do is what I do with Yemanja: pay attention. These two acts allow me to invoke silence as an assurance to the mother and baby that no matter what happens, my primary obligation is to them. Birth is an initiation for all involved and my silence is a container into which secrets spill but do not pass. It is my contract with the divine creators of the child to be born.

After listening and paying attention, I breathe with the body in front of me. Synchronizing my breathing with the mother-to-be allows me to sense subtle and overt changes in her being and allows us to communicate with each other when words are not possible. It will be the changes in the mother's breath during labour and the postpartum period that will guide me towards what she and the baby may need and what I need to do. It will be this breath that invites me to place my hand behind her back, on her hand, the nape of her neck.[33] It will be this breath that gives me permission to look directly into her eyes to let her know that she may place the weight of her body on my own and that my eyes will remain on her no matter what emotion she expresses or what happens around us.

It is a gift to touch another woman's body when another life rests within it. It is a humbling act of love to do this when that life is journeying towards our world. Like all transitions, birth is dirty and messy, violent even. It forces the mother to reveal parts of herself and bodily functions that she would never do willingly and to do so without apparent shame or apology. It forces me to witness it all with compassion reserved only for this event. Therefore, after committing to breathing with the mother, the next powerful thing I can do as a doula is to not turn away from the vomit, blood, excrement, snot, or tears that are essential parts of birth. In other words, I must not be afraid of the elements of life.

As a doula and an *egungun* priest, I have come to understand that life and death are inescapable components of our lives. Although the circumstances that bring us to these points vary and can be drastically different due to racial, cultural, economic, and social contexts, in the beginning and the end, they remind us that becoming and staying human are difficult tasks for all who undertake it. In the middle of the Atlantic Ocean, in the womb that is Yemanja, life and death are contained in such a profoundly obvious way that while swimming on a hot day, you might miss that fact. Seaweed mingles with dying fish. Shells crumble into sand. Salt water washes away skin. The tide carries away waste from other bathers. What does it mean to be inside the mother who creates and destroys in the same breath or wave? At the very least, it implies that the Yoruba worldview of motherhood and mothering is complicated: creation is often born out of destruction.

To swim in the ocean is to understand that Yemanja is the mother who fashions the greatest work of art: the child (Oyewumi 232-235). My approach to birthing, then, is a Yoruba-based one in which "the art of motherhood" is literal: the mother is responsible for shaping and crafting, if you will, new life by methods and manners unknown to me. Her materials are her own blood, muscle, sinews, thoughts, and spirit. Father and family are an integral part of the how and why the child is being brought into the world. However, it is the body of the mother in which the child waiting to be born lives and from which she or he receives nourishment.

It will be this body to which the child turns for sustenance first. This "matricentric" approach to birthing is one of the important factors that define my doula relationship with the mother and the way I approach "mothernity," or mothering (Diakite 62).

To enter the water, Yemanja, and to call on her is to challenge worldwide the concept of the "good mother," *the* one against whom all women are judged and some are found lacking. Like all the Yoruba *orisa*, Yemanja is more than what she appears to be and nothing we can comprehend. She is the mother who creates sharks and goldfish, who drowns coasts and reshapes shorelines. She is the mother who feeds her children, even as they destroy her. If one of the Great Mothers contains these contrasts within her, who am I to judge another woman as she learns how to become and be a mother?

As I learn more about what it means to be a doula, I have given gratitude to the Mother of Fishes. In her ever-changing perfection is mirrored the reality of my life and the life of other women. We struggle with light and shadow. My task as a doula is not to valorize one over the other. Perhaps it is to help the mother make way for both by guiding her as she digs deep into one more breath, one more push, to demonstrate to her that power is often found in the darkest corner of our spirits. It is here women have learned to tuck away the "super" and "wonder" part of themselves. As a healer, I know that what is hidden is not always "bad." Sometimes what is hidden in the dark is the secret key to our unfolding.

While caring for the living, I am not as far away as I thought from caring for the ancestors. In fact, choosing the doula path has made it possible to appreciate even more how the womb is a doorway to a place where the ancestors wait. According to holistic women's healthcare visionary and physical therapist Tami Lynn Kent, women carry the doorway to this place within the womb. "The womb," she writes, "is the connection to the spirit realm from which all spirits enter" (Kent 103). The womb, like the ocean, holds all possibility and history, making the mother not only the artist of life but also its primary archive and archivist.

From a Yoruba-based perspective, and maybe even an African-based one, becoming human is a multi-dimensional community venture steeped in the creation of worlds within worlds. During the birthing process, one of the final powerful things that I can do as a doula is to make certain that the mother knows before labour, during labour, and postpartum that her entire being is part of a community that holds her bodies in sacred time and space as she performs the most magnificent of miracles: birth. As a doula, I have been given the opportunity to know both the energetic and human bodies of the women I serve in ways that are at times more intimate than the ways I know my own body. I have been given the chance to know life and death as they greet each other in the only place of the human body that has yet to be understood by scientists and that will remain liminal, no matter how many times spirit becomes flesh. How I have found myself here is not the question at all. Clearly, I have been walking towards this path for a long time without knowing it; I have been passing through the realms of the ancestors to get to the doorway. Yemanja's waters flow through the doorway: Life before and after death.

ENDNOTES

[1]The *orisas* to whom one is initiated or to whom one has primary obligations are often referred and deferred to as "mother" and "father." The influence on a devotee's life is spoken of in terms of how they teach, shape, provide for, and/or discipline him or her.
[2]In fact, the first time I asked for an image of a Black Yemanja in Salvador da Bahia, the response I received was that such an image did not exist.
[3]I touch her belly only when the child waiting to be born invites me to do so.

WORKS CITED

Diakite, Dianne M. Stewart. "'Matricentric' Foundations of African Women's Religious Practices of Peacebuilding, Sustainability and Social Change." *Bulletin of Ecumenical Theology* 25 (2013): 62. Print.

Jones, Joni L. "Yoruba Diasporic Performance: The Case for a Spiritually – and Aesthetically – Based Diaspora." *Orisa: Yoruba*

Gods and Spiritual Identity in Africa and the Diaspora. Eds. Falola, Toyin and Ann Genova. Trenton: Africa World Press, 2005. 325-326. Print.

Kent, Tami Lynn. "The Spirit Door." *We'Moon 2013: Gaia Rhythms for Womyn.* Wolf Creek: Mother Tongue Ink, 2013. 103. Print.

Oyewumi, Oyeronke. "Beyond Gendercentric Models: Restoring Motherhood to Yoruba Discourses of Art and Aesthetics." *Gender Epistemologies in Africa: Gendering Traditions, Spaces, Social Institutions, and Identities.* Ed. Oyeronke Oyewumi. New York: Palgrave Macmillan, 2011. 223-238. Print.

Perez, Elizabeth. "Nobody's Mammy: Yemaya as Fierce Fore-mother in Afro-Cuban Religions." *Yemoja: Gender, Sexuality, and Creativity in the Latina/O and Afro-Atlantic Diasporas.* Eds. Solimar Otero and Toyin Falola. New York: SUNY Press, 2013. 9-41. Print.

United States Department of Commerce. United States Census Bureau. "Bloomington City, Indiana." *American FactFinder.* United States Census Bureau. 1 July 2010. Web. 30 Aug. 2014.

8.
"What Kind of Doula Are You?"

Birth Doulas, Multiple Moralities, and the Processes and Politics of "Ethical Becoming"

NICOLE C. GALLICCHIO

Every woman wants to be mothered by the 'The Infinite Breast,' to be thoroughly nurtured. And women in labor are vulnerable... even infantile. They really want to give their power away, and it is really hard for doulas to not just blindly accept that power.
—Virginia Grelling, birth doula and doula instructor

WHEN I FIRST EMBARKED ON my graduate studies, I was interested primarily in mothers: specifically, women's psychological transition to motherhood. It was as a research assistant for the University of Chicago Doula Project that I first heard about doulas, and my attention was irreversibly captured (Hans et al.). I became interested in birth doulas' inner lives, their ideas about and experiences with birth and caregiving, activism and authority, and how these informed their caregiving and expertise over time. To explore these issues in greater depth for my PhD research, I conducted an ethnographic study on birth doulas based primarily in the Northwest United States over a span of five years, from 2003 to 2008. I chose Pacific City and the surrounding region as my primary field site because of its rich wealth of educational opportunities for doulas and its "doula-friendly" reputation, with its primary doula training organization consistently striving to modernize and meet the needs of the doulas in the community and of families seeking doula care.[1] This time period marked a dynamic shift in the ideological environments surrounding reproductive activism. My dissertation research, therefore, ultimately focused on individual doulas' struggles to align their own complicated relationships to power and authority as well as their ideologies and ideals about birth with changing ideas within the larger doula movement around childbirth. I sought to complexify the doula role within this process by looking at contradictions, limitations, and negotiations that doulas experienced as they moved from "learning" to "doing."

In keeping with the findings of other doula researchers (see for example, Morton and Clift; Gilliland), I observed that as the new doulas in Pacific City moved from "learning" to "doing," they experienced profound highs and lows, which in many cases led to burnout or compassion fatigue. Over time, however, I found that those who continued their doula work developed (with the aid of more experienced doulas) creative ways to navigate the system, finding pockets of micropower within environments wherein they had initially felt powerless, and finding that they could, in fact, effect positive change on behalf of their clients. These pockets of micro-power lay within doulas' liminal status as institutional outsiders, their emotional connection with their clients, their authoritative knowledge, and their ability to read the emotional temperature of the birth room, all of which enabled doulas to enact strategies in service of their clients. As newer doulas became more agential in their practices, the risk that they would *over*power rather than *em*power their clients, inadvertently reproducing the very bio-medical power structure that they sought to contravene, became a real possibility. It is this issue, or rather, the doula community's response to this issue, that I explore in this chapter.

Within a few months of beginning my fieldwork, I grew curious about the emphasis placed by the doula community on self-ex-ploration throughout the formal and informal (i.e., scripted and unscripted) learning process. I observed an intriguing Durkheimian feedback loop between the community and the individual doulas as each worked to find the balance between ideology and prac-tice. At the heart of this seemed to be a kind of moral imperative that I could not quite grasp: I began focusing on what it meant to be a "good" doula as understood by individual doulas and their communities and on how both subjective positions affect the de-velopmental processes of individual doulas and their caregiving.

What I found was that it was based more on a morality- and ethics-driven assessment than on skill or outcomes: for the doulas in Pacific City, being a good doula was more about how to maintain and effectively balance a strong commitment to multiple realities and ideological frames in their caregiving than about their quantitative outcomes (i.e., their statistical track record with regards to Caesarean sections, epidurals, labour duration, and breastfeeding), number of births "under their belt," credentials amassed, community involvement, or their ability to perform a decent double-hip squeeze. Thus, it wasn't so much mastery of a certain set of skills that marked doulas as "good" in the eyes of their peers, nor did being good correspond with specific organizational loyalties or birth philosophies. Instead, what corresponded to being a good doula was something much more subtle and intangible: it was a kind of mastery over themselves, a self-awareness of themselves within and through the work, that garnered them the respect of the doula community.[2]

I observed several conversations between board members of two different certifying organizations in Pacific City about three different doulas, each of whom had applied for certification but were felt by some board members to be "dangerous." They were vouched for by other board members who said that although they may indeed be "dangerous," they were "good" doulas. Their politics and activism around childbirth reform made the board members nervous, particularly in light of recent "turf wars" between doulas and hospital staff in the region: in the birth room, however, they were able to put all of that aside and focus on the needs of their clients. Thus, it seemed that to be a good doula one needed to be able to authentically engage with, embody, and inhabit multiple (and even oppositional) subjectivities. Central to this ability was what I came to understand as the doula's development of an "expertise of the self," an expertise that would help circumvent the potential for a client to become an inadvertent pawn in a doula's power struggle with individual care providers or a general system of care. This "expertise of the self" encompassed the doulas' spiritual, corporeal, emotional, and psychological selves, including divergent ever-changing ideas about their own personhood.

Introductory doula trainings introduced the importance of developing this "expertise of the self" through a set of exercises designed to help students clarify why they were drawn to the work, and the ways in which these motivations might influence their caregiving: the ubiquitous "birth art" exercise, where students were given a piece of paper and markers and asked to illustrate their ideal birth; the word association exercise, where students free-associated with the word "birth" to elucidate hidden biases; and the "What Kind Of Doula Are You?" questionnaire, which the students were expected to fill out before the training and then after to see if their scores had changed. The doula instructors I interviewed, however, felt that these exercises, while important, were really more a kind of lip-service towards the goal of promoting truly ethical care. In effect, incorporated as they were into a massive, rushed process[3] of information distribution, these exercises did little to accurately assess whether or not a student would in fact become a "good" doula or provide the direction needed to initiate that process. This direction, I soon learned, was found not so much in the doula's formal pedagogical process but in the informal (and arguably more important) educational landscape of the doula community, within which a novice Pacific City doula was sure to find herself.

The importance of having the support of a doula community was emphasized time and again throughout my fieldwork; conversely, the lack of one was commonly mentioned as an obstacle to continued practice, and more than one doula was fearful of being "blacklisted." The doula community was therefore both a tremendous source of social support and a powerful pull toward social conformity. This dynamic was made most visible in the subtle but explicit social critique within the doula community around those doulas who were thought to lack self-awareness around themselves and their work. More experienced doulas regularly encouraged newer doulas to reflect on what might be at the root of any intense emotions that they might be feeling around birth, whether negative or positive: any emotion attached to a birth and that seemed to have a certain amount of pull to it was seen as fodder for examination. As a doula who invited me to apprentice with her for a birth told me over pizza one night during our post-birth debrief: "Doing this work cuts to the heart of what makes us human, and it can trigger a lot of unresolved stuff that you have to identify so that you can leave that birth baggage at the door when you enter a birth room." The phrase "birth baggage" was one that I heard repeated throughout the course of this study, and it was often invoked when a doula was experiencing intense emotions around her practice (whether positive or negative).

The birth doula community's emphasis on the development of self-awareness and self-knowledge as a fundamental part of the doula's education was informed by multiple influences: their beliefs about birth, power, the paradoxical relationship between a client's perceived vulnerability and her intrinsic strength; the potential impact of their own histories; and their understanding of their roles and ethical responsibility to their clients. As a beloved and well-respected doula from a neighbouring town, explained:

> Because this work draws certain kinds of women to it, there is a need for doulas to really think about why we're here. There are the saviour doulas who want to save their clients from having the kinds of traumatic experiences that happened to them, there are the activist doulas, and those who have a bone to pick with authority figures, and there are those who use births as a form of therapy—you can see those doulas coming from a mile away. And then there's the doula who just wants to take care of everyone because underneath it all she needs to be needed.

Some doulas in Pacific City were perceived by others as being too attached to the romance and drama of childbirth to be able to be fully present and responsibly attentive to a labouring woman's needs, while others were seen as being too rigid in their ideas about birth, which went against the flexible and fluid sense of self that doulas were expected to embrace in order to remain open to changing ideas and ideals. Thus "birth baggage" and the moral necessity of working through it represent the belief that a doula cannot truly provide sound, ethical care unless the doula's autonomy comes with a self-awareness capable of preserving her focus on the client (and her responsibilities to the client's needs). In this way, "dealing with your birth baggage" served as a kind of metaphorical and descriptive social script for Pacific City doulas to internalize, reflect on, and then ultimately enact in their practices, because a doula who had not successfully "dealt with her birth baggage" could not be a "good" doula. Doing so was critical with regards to one's moral standing within the doula community.

It became clear too that although the birth doula's subjective experience of becoming "good" was linked with her development of practical and pragmatic know-how, it was principally about self-discovery.[4] Opportunities to undertake this "study of the self" were worked into the fabric of the doula's (formal and informal) pedagogical landscape: examples included "re-birthing" workshops in which one's birth could be reenacted via hypnosis or external stimuli (e.g., participants progress through a "birth canal" of pillows) as a means of accessing "birth memories" stored in the body on a cellular level; doula-specific psychotherapy; study groups who met weekly to work through exercise books designed to identify and process subconscious "birth tigers;"[5] retreats, sweat lodges, and sharing circles; and numerous opportunities to get to know one's own body in intimate detail, for example through experiential learning in the form of vaginal exams, or mapping one's pelvic region at a "Pink Kit party." It was expected that through this process doulas would eventually master an "expertise of the self," specifically practices of self-awareness and self-regulation seen as keeping the doula's attention and care focused on the needs of the birthing woman.

Participating in the kinds of classes and undertakings described above (i.e., those meant to help doulas address their "birth baggage") over the span of several months or years helped doulas to feel as if they were taking the necessary steps to safeguard against being distracted from a focus on the mother by an alternate agenda of providing self-care. It was through this process, therefore, that doulas felt they could provide compassionate, emotionally engaged, and *ethical* care; this required that they respond effectively to the emotional and physical needs of individual clients regardless of whether or not they were aligned with the doulas' own moral or ideological commitments. In other words, the process of cultivating an "expertise of the self" provided doulas a way to deal with expectational disconnect and dissonance, and those tensions created when pragmatic concerns conflict with and by necessity supplant prior ideological commitments. Further, I believe the process of becoming a "good" doula helped doulas adjust to providing care in a far more complex social reality than trainings and predominant rhetoric surrounding doulas and doula support suggest. In this way, too, were they able to transcend such scripted binaries as home-hospital and natural-medical and focus on those elements of the birth experience that contribute to maternal emotional well-being and that, though contextually dependent, were well within the doula's purview. Developing this "expertise of the self" around—rather than through—the work of the doula allowed doulas to figure out for themselves how to navigate that ambiguous and amorphous line between being agential and pushing an agenda, between empowering and overpowering, and to learn how to support without supplanting.

Pacific City doulas enthusiastically embraced this kind of self-exploration, and even very new doulas did not wait until experienced doulas suggested to them that they embark on this process. In fact, most were quickly and actively engaged in efforts to clarify their positioning, due, I believe, to an unarticulated but very real concern about the possibility of subconsciously abusing their own power vis-à-vis their client.[6] The most frequent and visible efforts were around scope of practice clarification. Scope of practice debates, which generally developed out of questions posed by novice doulas seeking guidance, were highly polarizing and generally resulted in less clarity and more confusion about where a doula's ethical parameters lay. Doula mentors often took the "do as I say, not as I do" approach to explaining to questioning apprentices why they (the mentors) performed a manoeuvre, used a specific herb, or advised a course of action that was "officially" deemed to be outside the doula scope of practice. Many of the doulas had received training (and often certification) in other skillsets that were largely perceived to be outside the doula scope of practice (such as prenatal massage, aromatherapy, or acupressure). This was known in the doula community as "wearing a lot of hats"; knowing which "hat" was ethically appropriate at any given time was challenging, particularly when a doula felt that "just" wearing her "doula hat" limited her ability to fully support her client.

The challenge of delineating parameters around the doula role extended beyond scope of practice discussions. I observed, for example, two different doula communities launch outreach efforts at local hospitals that ultimately sputtered into anger, inaction, and ineffective silence over disagreements about the contents of a single-page informational handout, the stated but problematic goal of which was to detail what it is the doula would and would not do at each birth. Further, there was no one "type" of doula care to establish parameters around, with many different kinds of labour-support companions bearing the "doula" designation: for example, hospital-based doulas, community-based doulas, homebirth doulas, abortion doulas, doulas specializing in teen births, "radical" doulas, doulas based in prisons, "death" (hospice) doulas, and doulas volunteering for military personnel, all of whom learned a wide range of skill sets, with their own distinctive trainings and (usually) their own distinct objectives.

Further complicating matters were increasing tensions between changing ideas within the movement about what constituted an optimal birth and the underlying ideological frames that the doulas in this study still subscribed to. For instance, "natural childbirth" as a foundational ideology became something of an ideological grab bag over the course of my fieldwork. In Pacific City, as elsewhere, social movement rhetoric around childbirth was shifting from "natural birth" to "informed birth" with a focus on "choice," which reflected the recognition by those within the natural childbirth movement that women's individual circumstances needed to be taken into account (Bledsoe and Scherrer). However, although "informed choice" is arguably more equitable and universal than the "natural birth" ideal and can result in greater maternal autonomy, both linguistic components ("informed" and "choice") are complex culturally and socially loaded terms. Additionally, some have argued that the illusion of choice, and therefore the illusion of autonomy, keeps mothers (and their doulas) complicit within an oppressive and dehumanized system (Simonds et al.). Thus, even when Pacific City doulas succeeded in aligning themselves with the ideal of "informed choice" in childbirth, they inadvertently got caught up in the horns of race and class politics, particularly as they related to healthcare and perceptions of "deservedness,"[7] and the doula's own implicit assumptions and biases.

At this time, there was increasing focus on other problematic words that had historically been scripted into the doula role and that remained fully entrenched in movement discourse. "Empowerment" and "advocacy," for example,[8] were two words that many Pacific City doulas used as foundational tenets but that were sources of tremendous frustration for new doulas working to clarify the ethical ambiguities between their socially scripted roles and their scopes of practice. Indeed, during my fieldwork, the Pacific City-based regional arm of a national doula organization ultimately decided to omit the word "advocacy" from its "What Is A Doula?" position paper because, I was told, "the ambiguity around the word makes it too easy for doulas to overstep their bounds." A large doula cooperative from a nearby town removed all "empowerment"-related words from its mission statement for similar reasons. Despite (or perhaps further confused by) these kinds of organizational responses, however, the lack of clarity and resultant confusion remained in the community and within the individual doulas themselves.

Amid this confusion, new doulas continued to inadvertently create expectations for, and be hypervigilant around, producing a very specific kind of birth experience for their clients, predicated on a narrow set of beliefs about what constitutes an optimal birth and a perfect birthing environment. In other words, moving from "learning" to "doing" without recognition that the ideal of the empowered, informed, and autonomous birthing woman might preclude, and potentially eclipse, the ideals that the birthing woman herself may subscribe to. However, as they developed into their roles, moving from ideology into practice and becoming more fully engaged in what it means—philosophically, experientially, ethically, and practically—to care for their clients, I observed novice doulas' increasing awareness around these kinds of issues: specifically a growing internalized concern that they themselves might be contributing to those same kinds of structural power imbalances that they believed interfered with the potential for "true informed choice" in childbirth.

An additional complicating factor in delineating for a novice doula the "do's and don'ts" of ethical practice was a notable re-sistance within the community towards open discussion around doulas and their power. Despite the pride with which Pacific City doulas spoke about the power-*full* management strategies that they employed in the birth room in service to their clients, they had a complicated and ambivalent relationship with their own power.[9] Aside from a handful of outspoken doulas like Virginia Grelling (quoted above), there was a noticeable dearth of explicit discourse about doulas' power, particularly about the potential for power imbalances between the doula and her client: the discussion was more often focused around how to manage the power imbalances between the doula and the other members of the birth team, be-tween the labouring woman and her nurse, doctor, or midwife, or even between the doula-mother dyad and institutional structures. I believe that this resistance to conversations about power within the mother-doula relationship arose in large part because doulas found it profoundly difficult to open themselves to the possibility that they might inadvertently be contributing to the same kinds of structural abuse they worked so hard to contravene.

Novice doulas seemed to experience the relative silence on this issue as problematic for the confusion it revealed and instilled about the ethical parameters of a doula's use of power (given her complicated positioning between a "vulnerable" mother on the one hand and "dangerous" institutional practices on the other). Thus although "birth baggage" served as a helpful framework for doulas, helping to foster their pursuit of a kind of self-mastery from which they would experience greater internal and external coherence,[10] I would argue that it in fact represents something much more than that. It was through the process of "turning inward" and developing self-awareness, specifically around her own moral positioning, that the doula was able to begin complexifying her relationship to her own power, particularly vis-à-vis her client. From this vantage point, we can understand this emphasis on an "expertise of the self" as an integral part of the doula's develop-ment as a kind of organic, communal "check" within the system, given that the work of the doula exists in a liminal, inchoate space between social movement and legitimized profession.

The reality facing the doula in Pacific City mirrored the fragmented state of the national doula landscape. For instance, national, regional, and local training and/or certification organizations as well as local doula support groups and cooperatives all had mission statements of their own. And although the training and certification organizations had standards or scopes of practice doulas were supposed to abide by, each organization had its own. There was no apparent system in place to address the fact that the organization(s) with which a doula trained and the organization(s) with which a doula certified were not always the same. In addition, there were many doulas in Pacific City who opted out of the certification process entirely for financial, political, or other reasons. Given the lack of coherence in formal structures and intra- and inter-organizational politics on both a regional and national scale, and the absence of a consistent formalized system of "checks and balances" to offset the potential for doulas' (inadvertent) abuse of power vis-à-vis their clients, the only potential regulating body was that of the larger doula community in and around Pacific City, with its tremendous social pull.[11] It was through emphasizing the importance of an "expertise of the self" that this community sanctioned what constitutes a "good" doula and thereby exercised its informal authority, however imperfectly, to regulate the ethics of individual doula care.

The doula movement nationally, as in Pacific City, is still marked by struggles of morally infused meaning-making around issues relating to pregnant women, the socio-politics of reproduction in the United States, power and knowledge, consumers and healthcare consumption, the act of childbirth itself, the birthing body, and the woman herself (as both a part of and distinct from her physiological state). If the doulas in this study are indicative, reconciling these disparate meanings ultimately becomes the doula's primary struggle in what Faubion describes as the "process of ethical becoming." Further, amid this backdrop of reproductive politics and the shifting goals and rhetoric of the movement, the doula's client herself, as an experiencing subject —not just as The Patient, The Birthing Body, or The Mother—can be too easily overshadowed. In this way, "the woman in the body" can too easily get lost (Martin). However, by staying attuned to the complexity and intricacy of individual doulas' inner lives as they learn to navigate increasingly complex spheres of expertise and education, we can observe how they struggle to identify and stay true to the elusive moral heart of the work of the doula, to ultimately get (back) to truly woman-centred care. In Pacific City, doulas who succeeded in this endeavour did so by learning how to disengage from their own emotional investment and engage with the mothers' emotional experience as it unfolded. Being a "good" doula, therefore, was ultimately the ability to authentically embody and enact an ethic of care that centres around the individual women at the focus of the doulas' caregiving, taking into account their specific needs and contexts, and *not* around a generic "essential" birthing woman or around an activist agenda for changing the culture of birth in the United States.

Self-work was seen to be intrinsic to this process, and it was made all the more important by birth room politics and the paradoxical and problematic issues of power at work in the mother-doula relationship. Although doula-client power imbalances were rarely explicitly discussed, I came to understand that the emphasis on this inward turn, towards an "expertise of the self," dominated the doulas' educational landscape because it functioned as a kind of organic response to this risk potential from within the doula community. This response—propelled in part by a pull toward social conformity because of increasingly politicized "turf wars," professionalization tensions, a lack of consensus around the doula role and the absence of a comprehensive organizational structure— had more to do with the moral questions and ethical commitments at the heart of the doula movement than on the birth team power dynamics than I had initially thought. In this way, doulas learned how to stay true to the underlying concern of the doula movement—using this push towards an "expertise of the self" to carry movement ideals through the complex political landscape of childbirth, across the Gordian knot of entangled personal and professional goals, and into the pragmatics of day-to-day practice.

ENDNOTES

[1]The doulas in this study mirrored the demographic profile of

doulas nationwide at the time (Lantz et al.): the majority were women, white, married or in domestic partnerships, with at least one child, some college education, and for most, doula work was not their sole source of income. As part of my fieldwork, I took introductory birth doula trainings with the four national doula training organizations that had trained the most doulas in and around Pacific City (DONA, CAPPA, ALACE, and Birthing From Within), observed several more DONA-sponsored birth doula and postpartum doula trainings, attended three births through a doula mentorship program in Pacific City, and in addition to these births, was a birth doula for ten women and a postpartum doula for five. I conducted formal and informal interviews with fifty birth doulas at various stages during their developmental process: some were community-based doulas, but most worked with volunteer programs, private pay clients, and clients on public assistance, as community-based doula programs in the area were just developing.
[2]Although they freely used the word "good," doulas in Pacific City rarely called another doula "bad," but were more likely to speak *around* the negative designation: for example, "she has some growing to do" or "she has some issues she needs to look at."
[3]Most of the introductory birth doula trainings I observed occurred over the span of two weekends, generally starting at 8:30 a.m. and ending around 5:30 p.m., with an hour's worth of breaks scattered throughout the day.
[4]Interestingly, "good" caring often appears to have a mirror effect on the care providers themselves, in their own lives (Abel and Nelson 5). Doulas related to me how they had become better listeners and therefore better friends since beginning doula work, took better care of their own bodies and mental health, were more patient and less authoritative with their children, more tolerant and less judgmental of people in their communities, more forgiving towards parents with whom they had difficult relationships, and perhaps most profoundly, less willing to tolerate physical and mental abuse from partners, family members, and bosses.
[5]"Birth tigers," from Pam England's *Birthing from Within: An Extraordinary Guide to Childbirth*, represent fears around childbirth and/or the transition to parenthood.
[6]A particularly illustrative example of the kinds of contradictory

contexts that gave rise to these concerns took place one spring weekend at a workshop on birth and trauma: on Saturday, we were told by the instructor (a revered doula and doula educator in the community): "Don't let your mother go past the point of suffering. Even if she *really* wants a natural birth, she doesn't need to be a hero, and suffering can cause serious psychological trauma after the birth. So when you see in her eyes that she has gone from pain to suffering that is when you need to broach the subject of pharmacological pain relief and help her accept it." The following day, however, a co-instructor (also a well-respected member of the doula community) emphasized the importance of "helping women get over the hump" of wanting pain medication: "If your mom is committed to an un-medicated birth but had a traumatic birth experience with her first baby, she might get stuck around the spot where she felt her body or her process 'failed' her the last time. Your job is to help her through that. You all know how when a mom gets to the point where she's saying 'I can't do it anymore!' and she starts asking for an epidural, you know she's getting close and it's your job to insist that she *can* do it, and just encourage her to keep going and to push past that place? It's the same thing. Don't let her give in! Tell her she can do it. When everyone else is telling her to give up, you're the one telling her she can keep going without [an epidural]. So she will be able to reach that goal because you're believing in her when she can't believe in herself."
[7]See Craven; Nelson and Popenoe; Nestel; and Lazarus for insightful, detailed discussions of ongoing race and class politics around childbirth.
[8]"Autonomy," is also a word laden with complex social meanings that can challenge both the giving and receiving of care (Ehrenberg).
[9]This ambivalence is not surprising for many reasons. For instance, when a doula is hired to help a woman achieve *any* birth-related goals, this arguably "legitimizes" the doula's management strategies within and around the birth. Furthermore, because these strategies are employed in service to the birthing woman (in most cases with her knowledge and consent) and because they are focused on the (usually institutional) hierarchical power structure *in situ*, critical attention is deflected away from the doula's own power (following Lock and Kaufert 20). Indeed, the challenges

for the doula around clarifying her power and position vis-à-vis her client has roots in the very origins of the "doula" moniker, which was derived from the ancient Greek word for the female servant of a woman and developed in its contemporary usage by anthropologist Dana Raphael's 1955 *The Tender Gift*. Two African American doulas I spoke with refused to use the word "doula" because of its slavery connotations and preferred instead to use the term "labour companion," but the majority of the (White) doulas in my study felt that the ancient Greek meaning was an apt descriptor as it emphasized the service-based nature of the work. Whether rooted in a belief that doula work was a form of "civic activity" (Glenn) and/or "morally special" (Meagher), theirs was less of an exploitative and more of a moral economy, in keeping with, or at least building on, the "service" ideology that many doulas in the community were attracted to. This dynamic was vividly illustrated by the discomfort many doulas, particularly those with less experience, felt about charging their clients' money. In this way, the typical doula-client relationship inverts the traditional power dynamics of other caregiving relationships, which are usually rooted in race and class (Boris and Parreñas). Thus, contradictions around doulas' authoritative knowledge and their "service"-oriented positioning vis-a-vis the client, together with the client's own expectation that her doula will be a proxy for her autonomy, agency, and authority, make power issues particularly difficult to parse out and assess.

[10]In other words, when doulas' ideals or moral commitments were at odds with professional goals or ethics, and when these were at odds with practical and pragmatic considerations.

[11]It is important to note that those doulas who did not successfully engage with this process were increasingly pushed out to the margins of the community: socially and professionally exiled, as it were, and ostracized from the community support that they desperately needed if they were to continue practising. A common trajectory these individuals followed was to choose to discontinue their birth doula practices but find related work they felt that they were better suited to (e.g., lactation consultant, perinatal nutrition counseling, or postpartum doula): they were generally warmly supported by the doula community in these choices.

WORKS CITED

Abel, Emily and Margaret Nelson, Eds. *Circles of Care: Work and Identity in Women's Lives*. Albany, NY: Suny Press, 1990. Print.

Bledsoe, Carolyn and Rachel Scherrer. "The Dialectics of Disruption: Paradoxes of Nature and Professionalism in Contemporary American Childbearing." *Reproductive Disruptions: Gender, Technology, and Ethics in the New Millennium*. Ed. Martha Inhorn. Oxford: Berghahn, 2007. 47-78. Print.

Boris, Eileen and Rhacel Salazar Parreñas. *Intimate Labors: Cultures, Technologies, and the Politics of Care*. Stanford: Stanford University Press, 2010. Print.

Craven, Christa. *Pushing for Midwives: Homebirth Mothers and the Reproductive Rights Movement*. Philadelphia: Temple University Press, 2010. Print.

Ehrenberg, Alain. *The Weariness of the Self: Diagnosing the History of Depression in the Contemporary Age*. Montreal: McGill-Queen's University Press, 2009. Print.

England, Pamela and Robert Horowitz. *Birthing from Within: An Extraordinary Guide to Childbirth*. Albuquerque: Partera Press, 1998. Print.

Faubion, James. *An Anthropology of Ethics*. New York: Cambridge University Press, 2011. Print.

Gilliland, Amy. "From Novice To Expert: A Series of Five Articles", *International Doula*, publication of DONA International. Autumn 2007-Winter 2008; reprinted as e-book, June 2009. Print.

Glenn, Evelyn. "Creating a Caring Society." *Contemporary Sociology* 29.1 (2000): 84-94. Print.

Hans, Sydney, et al. "Promoting Positive Mother-Infant Relationships: A Randomized Trial of Community Doula Support For Young Mothers." *Infant Mental Health Journal* 34.5 (2013): 446-457. Print.

Lantz, Paula et al. "Doulas as Childbirth Paraprofessionals: Results from a National Survey." *Women's Health Issues* 15.3 (2005): 109-116. Print.

Lazarus, Ellen. "What Do Women Want? Issues of Choice, Control, and Class in Contemporary American Childbirth." *Childbirth and Authoritative Knowledge: Cross-Cultural Perspectives*. Eds.

Robbie Davis-Floyd and Carolyn Sargent. Berkeley: University of California Press, 1997.132-158. Print.

Lock, Margaret and Patricia Kaufert. "Introduction." *Pragmatic Women and Body Politics*. Eds. Margaret Lock and Patricia Kaufert. London: Cambridge University Press, 1998. 1-27. Print.

Martin, Emily. *The Woman in The Body*. Boston: Beacon Street Press, 2001. Print.

Meagher, Gabrielle. "Is it Wrong to Pay for Housework?" *Hypatia: A Journal of Feminist Philosophy* 17.1 (2002): 52-66. Print.

Morton, Christine and Elayne Clift. *Birth Ambassadors: Doulas and the Re-emergence of Woman-Supported Birth in America*. Amarillo, TX: Praeclarus Press, 2014. Print.

Nelson, Margaret and Rebecca Popenoe. "Looking Within: Race, Class, and Birth." *Birth By Design: Pregnancy, Maternity Care, and Midwifery in North America and Europe*. Eds. Raymond DeVries et al. New York: Routledge, 2001. 87-114. Print.

Nestel, Sheryl. "Delivering Subjects: Race, Space, and the Emergence of Legalized Midwifery in Canada." *Canadian Journal of Law and Society* 15.2 (2000): 187-215. Print.

Raphael, Dana. *The Tender Gift*. New York: Schocken Books, 1955. Print.

Simonds, Wendy et al. *Laboring On: Birth in Transition in the United States*. London: Routledge, 2007. Print.

9.
"My Role Is to Walk the Tightrope"

Doulas and Intimacy

ANGELA N. CASTAÑEDA AND JULIE JOHNSON SEARCY

THIS RESEARCH FOCUSES ON THE multiple ways bodies are materialized through the intimate practices of *doulaing* and birthing. In this paper, we are interested in addressing three main questions: What are the implications of the intimate labour performed by doulas? More specifically, how does mothering performed by doulas craft particular understandings of birthing bodies? And how might viewing these bodies as active and fluid material realities challenge existing practices as forms of embodied resistance?

The work that doulas do represents a complex and multidimensional form of intimate labour. Medical anthropologist Dana Raphael is credited with applying the word doula when describing the importance of "mothering the mother" during the fourth trimester to increase successful breastfeeding results. Today, much of this "mothering" takes place in institutionalized settings with the overwhelming majority of women in the United States giving birth in hospitals. We are interested in exploring intimate labour as a useful category of analysis to understand the role of doulas, described by some as "fourth-class citizens," within institutional birth settings that privilege the use of clinical knowledge to standardize the birthing body (Norman and Rothman 267). Doulas simultaneously use the fluidity of their own bodies to cross the border from an intimate to an institutional setting while they also highlight the importance of a personalized birthing body. We suggest that the kind of intimate labour undertaken by doulas provides opportunities for embodied resistance in response to homogenizing models of birth.

METHODS

The data collected for this project is grounded in ethnographic methods spanning two years, from 2012 to 2014. We focused our research on a small U.S. Midwestern town with a thriving doula community. Given the size and nature of this site, we changed the names of all participants to protect their identities. We used multiple modes of data collection, including semi-structured interviews, focus groups, online surveys, and content analysis of web-based material such as blogs. We conducted interviews with twenty-five doulas, sixteen labour and delivery nurses, four administrators, and six childbirth educators. In addition, we used participant observation and engaged with this community as practising birth and postpartum doulas for dozens of mothers and families. Ultimately, our work as anthropologists, doulas, and mothers involves traversing and negotiating intimate spaces where we find competing forms of knowledge involving the intimate labour performed by doulas.

INTIMATE: FROM THE LATIN *INTIMUS*,
MEANING VERY CLOSE, INNERMOST, OR DEEPEST

Doula work is often described as mothering the mother, and it emphasizes a physical, spiritual, and emotional connection between women. In all three of these categories, we find doulas working with labouring women in ways that require intimacy. Intimate labour, as Boris and Parreñas acknowledge, entails "bodily or emotional closeness, close observations of another and personal knowledge or information" (2). Doulas engage in multiple practices that "personalize" (Morton and Clift 122) and, in turn, produce intimate knowledge of a birthing body.

Doula work is not only physical but also gruelling. To provide continuous support during a birth, a doula commits to staying with the woman from the moment she calls requesting help until the baby is born and has successfully breastfed. This can mean three hours or three days. After walking away from a birth, a doula can be both emotionally and physically marked. Jane described her memory of one of her first births:

And then she went into labour and had her home birth. And it was a very intense birth. She had a shoulder distortion, and it was very very intense. She was on hands and knees when she was delivering, and she was holding onto me. I had bruises on my legs and arms from where she pushed so hard into me with her elbows and grabbed me with her arms.

Another doula recalled: "I thought I would use all the toys in my doula bag, but after attending a few births I realized that none of that was really important. It was just me, my body, that I used the most." The physical care doulas provide birthing women allows them access to intimate knowledge about birth and bodies. As they witness the physical act of birthing a baby, doulas also engage their own bodies in physical exertion. In these examples, doulas realized it was their own physical presence that provided the support and assistance for a woman in labour. And many doulas recalled the memory of births through their own bodies in the form of "bruises from a tight grip," "marks from an uncomfortable chair," or a "sore neck, back, and shoulders." Yet the physicality of doula work is balanced with an attention towards a "doula spirit" as well as towards the emotional state of both the doula and birthing mother.

In addition to the physical intensity of their work, doulas also identified birth as deeply processual; for them, birth itself was a transformative process for both the mother and the doula. Sometimes this process was spiritual in nature as Ruth shared:

[It was] the spiritual thing that brought me to [doula work], so I get the privilege of witnessing women go through a process that strips them of all those pretenses and gets them down to what's real and gets them to where they don't think they can do it, and they reach out and then they do it. And to me, I always say God drew me into doula work because he knew my faith needed regular renewal.

For Ruth, the process of birth and her work as a doula reflect a critical part of embodied care and mothering the mother. Other doulas identified moments of personal transformation with birth, as illustrated in Maria's response:

I was always terrified of childbirth myself since I was little because I thought it would be super painful ... also I was a victim of sexual abuse so that kind of played into it as well. But since becoming a doula, I have seen amazing things, and I just have no doubts in my mind about what my body is capable of, so for me personally it has been transformative in terms of my own confidence about birth.

The spiritual nature of doula work encompasses secular and sacred realms as doulas learn to negotiate their physical and emotional experiences with birth. As doulas attend to their own and birthing mothers' emotional and spiritual states, they recognize the diversity of experiences and realities that materialize during birth.

To provide continuous care to a labouring woman necessitates some degree of emotional connection and care, which flows between a labouring mother and doula. Both mothers and doulas emphasized building emotional attachments to one another. Mothers described this lasting relationship by calling their doula, "an important person in our family," and by describing their doula as "a permanent part of our lives." Most doulas also said that their relationships with clients extend past the postpartum visit, as one doula noted, "I keep in touch with all of my clients well beyond the birth. I don't think you can be at someone's birth and then just disappear from their life. My clients and I feel a connection that goes beyond what they've hired me to do." This relational work allows a doula to provide intimate support during birth.

In their work, doulas engage in intimate labour that relies on close observation to care for birthing women. Doulas work to cultivate trust with a labouring woman through their use of observation, continuous care, bodily upkeep, closeness, and touch. Doulas wipe foreheads, share supportive words, and hold hands with labouring women, and when they walk away from a woman and her newly delivered baby, they carry personal knowledge and information about that woman.

The work that doulas perform pushes the boundaries of intimate labour. In "Caring Everywhere," Viviana Zelizer identifies intimate labour as performed in four sites: "unpaid intimate care in intimate settings, unpaid intimate care in economic organizations, paid care in economic organizations, and paid care in intimate settings" (270). Doulas assist labouring women in intimate home settings and often transition to institutional spaces such as hospitals. Doula work means crossing the spaces Zelizer identifies as sites for intimate labour. In crossing these sites, doulas are required to embrace the liminal nature of their role.

LIMINAL: FROM LATIN *LĪMEN*, MEANING THRESHOLD

In one ethnographic moment, Lisa and I (JJS) sit in the warm sun of a coffee shop as she thoughtfully says, "I am trying to think about what's so ... different about this work and how to describe it." I am asking her about her work as a doula, work that she has been doing for almost a decade. She is in her mid-thirties and began work as a doula before she had children. Lisa has attended over one hundred births but has recently taken a break after the birth of her first daughter. She says:

> *I think it has to do with the way this profession defines boundaries. Being clear about what the doula-client relationship is and what the parameters of that are [is important]. I think that in any sort of caretaking helping profession [these boundaries are] really important because we are involved intimately in people's personal lives.*

Lisa points to a tension as she tries to articulate the kind of care provided by doulas. She describes the kind of intimate work doulas do: fielding phone calls at all hours of the night, seeing women in intimate spaces of their homes and bathrooms as a birth unfolds.

Doula work is intimate and liminal in nature. Doulas navigate boundaries while they work with labouring women, within their doula community, and with care providers.

Doulas and Mothers

Doulas are invited to become intimately involved in a pregnant woman's life by being present at a birth, yet this invitation is often attached to a contract with an expectation for payment at the end. Missy, a doula in this community, explained this relationship by noting, "Women often don't understand what they are paying for really. I mean, in addition to my actual doula services, I have to rearrange my life to be on call for them. And I feel like that's kind of the part that's hard to quantify in terms of money." Jane echoed this sentiment: "I really learned my lesson once when I rearranged my vacation schedule to be at a birth and then, they didn't call me. That was a real like, 'Oh, I see.' I took it more seriously than they did. That was the point in which I really felt like some trust had been broken." Trust is a key component in the working relationship between a labouring woman and her doula. One mother from our focus group shared the importance of this relationship:

My doula made me trust in my body and what was happening, and trust in the baby. There was this special moment during labour when I was already six centimeters open, but I felt disappointed, and I remember her saying to me, "Six centimeters is wonderful. Now you can take a shower, and it is going to go quickly from here." So my confidence was back, and after that I knew I could birth my baby because I felt it was my body's purpose. I was made to do this, and I did.

The intensity of the experience shared by doulas and labouring women translates into potentially permeable boundaries that doulas must take care to manage. Jane described this situation as a "dance" where she must honour who the labouring woman is and what she wants with her own knowledge as a birth worker:

While we're developing this relationship and bonding, we can't bond completely. She needs to keep her separateness ... she really needs to know as little as possible about me. And you can see it too, when it'll occur to her, "Oh, maybe I should ask you about yourself." And if I give anything but a short answer, she glazes over. Because really, she's not interested, and frankly she shouldn't be.

Because I need to be a projection screen, otherwise, she might try to please me or get me to like her, in a way that she changes what she wants to do. And that's not necessarily healthy for her.

Doulas often describe their work as "holding the space," their community as a "sisterhood ministry," and their presence at a birth as "an honoured guest." Yet doulas are also faced with pressure to legitimize their work via a process of professionalization that often conflicts with performing a doula spirit of unconditional support.

Doula Spirit and Doula Professionalism

The doula community itself is also a space where doulas find themselves navigating the boundaries between perceived degrees of professionalism within their practice. As doulas explained their work, they described two perceived competing logics: one influenced by embodied care and the other by a neoliberal market. We describe embodied care as a lived experience that is "relational, fluid and processual" (Jaye 41). This reflects what we heard from doulas who speak about their work in terms of a "doula spirit" that is performed, shared, and demonstrated through their interactions with mothers, fellow doulas, and other care providers. This form of care competes with a neoliberal market model in which individuals see themselves as sets of skills that need careful marketing (Gershon 539; Harvey 42). We return to Lisa, a doula who we heard from at the beginning of this section, as she discussed the importance of balancing boundaries in doula work:

Another problem about professionalism is walking the balance of honouring this work as important work that deserves financial compensation and respect and also honouring the emotional, spiritual intensity of it. And I feel like I see people swing both ways, where it's like this work is so amazing, and I'm so privileged to do it that I will just do it for free. And that doesn't honour the energy exchange that is required and that burns people out. Nobody can sustain that for very long, and on the flipside I've seen some doulas more recently who really want to do it as a job, and it lacks something deeper; ultimately it's a hard balance to strike.

The difficulty in balancing a doula spirit within an increasingly commercialized birth culture is echoed in Helen's observations:

[I find with] the business mind versus the mothering mind, there is a huge conflict. The conflict is why am I charging to do something women have been doing for thousands of years? It should just be a given, but I think the reason I'm charging is because the world has changed. And the birth culture has changed.

In their efforts to negotiate the two contrasting logics, doulas turn to professional organizations and marketing techniques to find spaces that help regulate and mediate the conflict of interest inherent in neoliberal alliances. As veteran doula Jane commented:

Drawing boundaries, getting certifications, putting a price on it, making contracts, and running [it] like a business, that's the entrepreneurial doula. And I feel like the entrepreneurial doula is more inclined to ask, "What's in it for me?" And this is not an illegitimate question, but if you foreground that enough you get into charging by the hour or getting into charging weird things, which might backfire depending on what the community is like or what the tone is where you practice.

Doulas navigate the boundaries within their own community as they undertake the intimate labour of balancing professionalization with the emotional and spiritual nature of the labour that they provide. Doulas have to think through how alignment with professional organizations will affect their relationships with clients. The decision to align with a professional organization also influences the experience of doulas within institutional settings.

Doulas and Care Providers
The intimacy involved with doula work is heightened as the

doula's role becomes more professionalized, and doulas are tasked with making smooth transitions in and out of institutional settings. Labour and delivery nurses are the care providers who interact the most with doulas, and unfortunately, the relationship between these birth workers is often one fraught with tension (Papagni and Buckner; Gilliland).

Doulas and nurses perform different kinds of intimate practices that render different material realities of the birthing body. Both doulas and nurses rely on close observation to care for birthing women. When nurses and doulas walk away from a woman and her newly delivered baby, they both carry personal knowledge and information about that woman through the work that they've performed. They both work to cultivate trust with a labouring woman through their use of close observation, bodily upkeep, closeness, and touch. However, the extent of this closeness and touch varies in terms of its acceptability, as one labour and delivery nurse wrote in her online survey, "The difficult doula borders on sexual abusive behaviours (in my opinion). Rubbing [the] patient in areas, not wearing gloves, constantly moaning with the patient for hours!"

Institutional knowledge and technological practices encourage nurses to see a birthing body as potentially dangerous. Courtney, a labour and delivery nurse, noted: "There are just two different ways to view the situation—one is from the nurse which views birth as a potential problem waiting to happen, and the other is from a doula who views birth as a natural process." Nurses are bound by professional and institutional rules and regulations that standardize the birthing body, and "At times it seems that [this] standardizing overwhelms [their] primary activity...." (Lampland and Star 10). In our research, we heard resentment and frustration from nurses when discussing the impact of this standardization. Courtney, sharing her experience as a nurse, stated:

I wanted to be the professional doula and take care of the mother, and you really can't do that because there is so much to do because of all the interventions, which are ridiculous. Moms and nurses are overwhelmed with the amount of things to do, starting IVs, charting, monitors, and if you have a lot going on or a problem, emotionally the moms fall out of the picture.

Courtney's description highlights how standardized institutional practices overshadow her ability to see past the surface layer of a birthing body. This use of clinical knowledge to standardize the birthing body further alienates doulas within the hospital and frames their role as "fourth-class citizens" (Norman and Rothman 267). A nurse's intimate labour produces a birthing body rooted in a technological frame, which is clearly situated in Robbie Davis-Floyd's technocratic model of birth. This emphasis on how "the institution is a more significant social unit than the individual" (483) was echoed by one of the doulas we interviewed who shared:

If I'm not in the room, then the nurse is never knocked out of her trance state to recognize that she is working with an individual, who might need something different than she thinks she does. If I'm not in the room, then the nurse just thinks she's a difficult patient instead of realizing she's a rape survivor and she has some special needs at the moment. Instead, what the nurse needs is for her people to just burst into the room and touch her without asking.

Within institutional spaces, the birthing body is read by nurses through technological measurements dictated by institutional policies. Nurses must manage the birthing body in this way, even as they often hope for more emotional closeness. The doula's presence highlights and makes visible the tension involved with intimate labour in an institutional setting. We argue that this tension comes from the different intimate labour performed by nurses and doulas, which in turn privileges a particular kind of birthing body. Within the liminal space occupied by doulas, they find opportunities for resistance and the creation of a more personalized birthing body.

RESISTANCE: FROM THE LATIN *RESISTERE*, MEANING TO MAKE A STAND AGAINST OR OPPOSE

In her article, "Surfacing the Body Interior," anthropologist Janelle

Taylor emphasizes that, "not only ideas but also material realities, including bodies, are in fact made and continually remade through practice" (744). She argues that "surfacing the body interior points toward the range of practices and processes that both materialize bodily surfaces as significant sites within broader orders, and surface that which lies hidden beneath them" (Taylor 742). In our research, we found this distinction with bodily surfaces useful in framing doula work as a form of embodied resistance.

Embodied resistance is rooted in the practices of doula care. Indeed, for Taylor,

> The body ... is not so much a thing as an -*ing*. That is, [it is] not simply the inert objects on which mind and culture perform their meaning making, [but instead] bodies take shape and take place through practices of all sorts: feeding, legislating, training ... and healing, among others. (745)

To this list we add doulaing, a practice that occupies liminal spaces where doulas move between private and institutional settings and perform intimate labour. As doulas labour, "embodied experiences intermix, and from/in this fluid boundary state, resistance to cultural scripts and emergent knowledge can potentially arise" (Lewiecki-Wilson and Cellio 2). Doulas build relationships with mothers and families, and their liminal position opens up the possibility for new meaning making.

How is surfacing the body interior linked to embodied resistance for doulas? The kind of labour doulas undertake gives them the ability to access knowledge from labouring bodies that others cannot because of the unique boundaries doulas traverse as they work. The practices that doulas undertake reveal material birthing bodies as well as "broader orders and the surfaces that lie beneath them" (Taylor 742). Doulas bring to maternity care an ability to view the labouring woman and her body through the lens of personalization. We argue that personalizing means materializing, uncovering, acknowledging, and respecting a birthing body.

Doulas cross boundaries to protect and support the fluid nature of a birthing body, which can be liberating for both the doula and mother. In moving between home and hospital, and from physical support to emotional support, doulas recognize the material reality and work of birth. Yet doulas also perform the role of educator or information provider, especially involving protection from negative forms of boundary crossing, such as misuse of authoritative knowledge or (mis)informed consent (Jordan; Rapp). For example, at one of the births that I (JJS) attended, I watched an obstetrician prepare to perform an episiotomy on a labouring woman without informing her. In prenatal visits with the couple, episiotomies were discussed and the mother made her preference against one very clearly. I discretely pointed out what was happening to the husband who questioned the obstetrician. The obstetrician, clearly annoyed, told the mother that she was "going to tear anyway" and needed his help. The mother told the doctor that she did not want his help and was able to avoid an episiotomy. In this instance, teaching and educating is a form of resistance for doulas. Because doulas engage in prenatal discussions and education before they enter the birth space, they are able to personalize birth in light of the preferences women and their partners express. As Jane noted, "It's tricky, because I'm an educator and education is always radicalizing." Jane recognizes that personalized birth is often perceived as radical, or at the very least an irritant to the depersonalized protocols of institutions.

Several mothers in our focus groups provided examples of how doulas personalize birth experiences while they engaged in resistance. Emily said, "We didn't even know what questions to ask. She [our doula] told us what questions to ask our OB and that sent the signal that we wanted less interventions." Sarah described her experience during labour, "At the hospital a group of trainee nurses came in and asked, 'Can we watch?' And I remember her [my doula] saying vehemently, 'No, you cannot. This is not a theatre.'" And after her daughter was born with breathing issues and taken to the nursery, Olivia recalled the role of her doula, "It was important to have the doula with me to keep me distracted and eventually get pissed off after they kept her [my daughter] from me, far longer than the optimal time to latch. Her knowing that it was time to get pissed off was really helpful."

Doulas engage in embodied resistance when they materialize

the birthing body as emotive and layered; a practice that conflicts with a more homogenized institutional birthing body as identified from a clinical gaze. Jane, a veteran and leader in this doula community, identified the difference between standardized and individualized care:

A culture that thinks it's good to have labour support is a culture that is making better births for women. Because this would mean we would no longer be one size fits all for births. It would be admitting that individual women want different things, whatever that is ... it's a mistake to think the that the very act of having someone in the room caring for emotions is not a radical act because the hospital doesn't give a shit about her emotions. They're concerned with did the baby come out and breath. Is she alive at the end? And is the baby alive? That's what they care about. And they should care about that. I don't mean to denigrate that at all. That's extremely important; however, it leads them to dismiss what [a labouring woman] is feeling.

Personalizing a birthing body is a process that highlights the relational nature inherent in doula work, and it emphasizes the intimate and liminal contexts within which doulas operate. These are characteristics of doulaing that open the door to embodied forms of resistance.

CONCLUSION

My role is to walk the tightrope.... It's living on the edge of the boundaries and that's what makes it [doula work] a powerful role, and the best births occur when the tension is held among all those things and something new emerges. That's the beauty of it. (Jane, doula)

The intimate labour performed by doulas privileges a particular form of knowledge that highlights the ways bodies materialize meaning. As doulas walk the tightrope, balancing boundaries between mothers, doulas, and care providers, they have access to multiple vistas. An exploration of the mothering doulas perform can serve as a space to understand the nuances of providing intimate care. Ideally, doulas engage in physical, spiritual, and emotional labour, treating each woman they work with as an individual who requires careful observation of her material body so that they can personalize their care for her. This intimate labour also means moving between relational and institutional boundaries as doulas follow the birthing body.

The different ways bodies are materialized for doulas demonstrate the importance of analyzing the practices involved with intimate labour. Practices, as defined by Sara Ruddick in her groundbreaking book *Maternal Thinking*, "are collective human activities distinguished by the aims that identify them and by the consequent demands made on practitioners committed to those aims" (13-14). The potential for doula practices rooted in intimate labour to personalize birth and challenge our current birth culture was shared by doula Lisa:

> *When I think about what messages I want little girls to hear about birth, I want them to hear that it was a lovely day, and that I felt wonderful that day. No matter what happens ... children are going to hear the tone and the emotion; they are not going to hear the details. Instead what matters are the feelings, and then if that's what they are growing up with [positive feelings] rather than fear, regret, and anxiety, then they are more likely to go into [birth] thinking that it is a positive experience, whatever choices they make.*

Lisa saw the intimate work of doulas as helping to produce a particular feeling around birth, in part because of the practices doulas undertake. In particular, doula practices privilege an emotive, layered, and personalized birthing body. Ultimately, doulas illustrate how bodies, as material realities, are shaped and reshaped. And as we investigate how doulas negotiate boundaries, we can find an alternative narrative to the popular narrative of what a birthing body is in our culture.

WORKS CITED

Boris, Eileen and Rhacel Salazar Parreñas. "Introduction." *Intimate Labors: Cultures, Technologies, and the Politics of Care.* Eds. Eileen Boris and Rhacel Salazar Parreñas. Stanford, CA: Stanford University Press, 2010. 1-17. Print.

Davis-Floyd, Robbie E. "The Technological Model of Birth." *Journal of American Folklore* 100.398 (1987): 479-495. Web. 11 Nov. 2014.

Gershon, Ilana. "Neoliberal Agency." *Current Anthropology* 52.4 (2011): 537-555.Web. 25 Feb. 2012.

Gilliland, Amy L. "Beyond Holding Hands: The Modern Role of the Professional Doula." *Journal of Obstetric, Gynecologic, & Neonatal Nursing* 31.6 (2002): 762-769. Web. 1 March 2012.

Harvey, David. *A Brief History of Neoliberalism.* Oxford: Oxford University Press, 2005. Print.

Jaye, Chrystal. "Talking around Embodiment: The Views of GPs Following Participation in Medical Anthropology Courses." *Medical Humanities* 30 (2004): 41-48. Web. 8 March 2012.

Jordan, Brigitte. "Authoritative Knowledge and Its Construction." *Childbirth and Authoritative Knowledge: Cross-Cultural Perspectives.* Eds. Robbie E. Davis-Floyd and Carolyn F. Sargent. Berkeley: University of California Press, 1997. 55-79. Print.

Lampland, Martha, and Susan Leigh Star, eds. *Standards and Their Stories: How Quantifying, Classifying, and Formalizing Practices Shape Everyday Life.* Cornell: Cornell University Press, 2009. Print.

Lewiecki-Wilson, Cynthia and Jen Cellio. "Introduction." *Disability and Mothering: Liminal Spaces of Embodied Knowledge.* Eds. Cynthia Lewiecki-Wilson and Jen Cellio. Syracuse, NY: Syracuse University Press, 2011. 1-15. Print.

Morton, Christine H. and Elayne Clift. *Birth Ambassadors: Doulas and the Re-emergence of Woman-Supported Birth in America.* Amarillo, TX: Praeclarus Press, 2014. Print.

Norman, Bari Meltzer and Barbara Katz Rothman. "The New Arrival: Labor Doulas and the Fragmentation of Midwifery and Caregiving." *Laboring on: Birth in transition in the United States.* Eds. Wendy Simonds, Barbara Katz Rothman, and Bari Meltzer

Norman. New York: Taylor & Francis, 2007. 251-282. Print.

Papagni, Karla, and Ellen Buckner. "Doula Support and Attitudes of Intrapartum Nurses: A Qualitative Study from the Patient's Perspective." *The Journal of Perinatal Education*15.1 (2006): 11-18. Web. 4 April 2012.

Raphael, Dana. *The Tender Gift: Breastfeeding.* Englewood Cliffs, NJ: Prentice-Hall, 1973. Print.

Rapp, Rayna. "Foreword." *Childbirth and Authoritative Knowledge: Cross-Cultural Perspectives.* Eds. Robbie E. Davis-Floyd, and Carolyn F. Sargent. Berkeley: University of California Press, 1997. xi-xii. Print.

Ruddick, Sara. *Maternal Thinking: Toward a Politics of Peace.* Boston: Beacon, 1989. Print.

Taylor, Janelle S. "Surfacing the Body Interior." *Annual Review of Anthropology* 34 (2005): 741-756. Web. 16 March 2012.

Zelizer, Viviana. "Caring Everywhere." *Intimate Labors: Cultures, Technologies, and the Politics of Care.* Eds. Eileen Boris and Rhacel Salazar Parreñas. Stanford, CA: Stanford University Press, 2010. 267-279. Print.

10.
Providing Boundaries
in Postpartum Doula Care

JACQUELINE KELLEHER

POSTPARTUM DOULA WORK IS LIFE. It offers experiences
that are gritty, expansive, and as diverse and wonderful as
the families we serve. It is not easy to plan for, as the doula
finds herself immersed in people's lives—in their homes, with their
families, their friends, their joys and challenges. Loss and grief,
relationship and identity struggles are as likely to be encountered
as excitement and a desire to learn and adapt. In order to define
our role as doulas, we must express our limits. In a position that
inherently knows no bounds, it is crucial that the individuals
providing the service also provide the boundaries.

As a postpartum doula, my role is unique. In fact, I'm hard
pressed to find another role as expansive and intimate. I am
in the home with the family for hours at a time, several days
a week, sometimes for as long as the first three months. There
is no one else there—no supervisor, no medical personnel. As a
doula, I am functioning on an island. The lack of a clinical care
provider is inherent, since healthy families with a new baby only
require the occasional checkup as determined by their baby's
doctor. That isolation does mean, however, that I am the primary professional voice in their lives. My voice is powerful and
matters to this family. My responsibility is to know my stuff. If
I am sharing information on matters such as infant feeding and
newborn needs and characteristics, I have to be certain that my
information is the most accurate available because to be honest,
there is no one who has my back or the back of the parents. In
our small, intimate worlds, we can all benefit from boundaries

to keep our interactions as healthy and as productive as possible.

Doulas provide anticipatory guidance. We know what may be coming next. While the parents are experts on their own family, as the doula, I am an expert on normal adjustment and the challenges that may arise within it. Doulas possess training, education, and with time, a wealth of experience. In the past twenty years, I have acquired hundreds of hours of classroom education focused on the childbearing year. After training as a childbirth educator, birth and postpartum doula, I studied the newborn through the Brazelton Institute and also became a certified lactation counsellor. I have facilitated thousands of hours of new parent groups. Between my experience as a doula and lactation counsellor, I have worked with hundreds of new families on a 1:1 basis. As a doula, I have been here before—very likely, many times. My clients have not. The onus is on me to chalk out the boundaries as I forge new client relationships and maintain those boundaries throughout our time together. These boundaries protect my clients, my family, and me. Boundaries are not always easy, but they are always necessary.

In my tenure as a postpartum doula, I have experienced a great variety of situations that held promise for either growth or challenging outcomes for all. These most often are innocuous—clients who are looking for primarily childcare (not my role) or house cleaning (not my role either). I quickly learned to clearly define my role and to develop the language and the skills to keep my clients and me focused on that of support, rather than doing for. Other situations have been more murky and challenging: the clients with their baby born morphine addicted who wanted me to feed the baby with the drug in the bottle as part of the weaning process (I required them to feed the baby); the parents who asked a doula friend to take their truck so that she would be able to get to them the next day despite a snowstorm; and the parents who used parenting strategies that evidence proves to be inappropriate and dangerous for a newborn. These are the situations in which the doula is acutely aware of her isolation with the family. There are no peers to bounce thoughts off at lunch; there is no supervisor to make sure that she makes the "correct" choice. This means that both my profession and I are responsible for upholding a certain standard within our work.

SEPARATE ROLES

I have been asked why I feel so strongly that postpartum doulas be mindful of boundaries at all times. To be clear, I believe that boundaries are a priority for all professions, including birth doulas. That said, I have ample experience in both types of doula work, and I have observed some distinctions. Birth doula work is linear. Although there can be many possible permutations of the birth doula experience, it always begins with a pregnant woman and ends with a baby on the outside. It is also limited by time—prenatal visits, the labour, a postpartum follow-up visit. The role is clearly defined and although the doula may keep in contact with the family afterward, the time that she spent actively as their birth doula has an inherent ending. Postpartum doula work is quite different. We may meet the clients prenatally or weeks after the birth of the baby. We may visit them only once or have more than fifty visits. There are no clinical personnel present. While the birth doula's role is linear, the role of the postpartum doula can feel more like a wagon wheel, with the doula in the centre. Her role can differ greatly from family to family—sometimes breastfeeding, sometimes integrating the baby with older siblings, sometimes helping a mother cope with depression, or sometimes working to connect the family with a community. And this can go on for months.

GETTING THERE

Before I can begin this process and enter my clients' home, I must first leave my own behind. More important than geography is the emotional act of shelving my roles of mother and partner, among other responsibilities. A big part of being able to do that is having a partner who understands my work and is supportive of my decision to entwine my time and energy and emotions with those of others. Doula work is different from other jobs. Supporting new families can be consuming. Triumphs and challenges remain in our minds—and often our phones and emails—long after we've returned home. My marriage, my home, and my children have all been shaped by doula work. Having worked as both a birth and postpartum doula beginning with three of our children, I have experienced a gamut of approaches and negotiations as we have moved through the changes in financial and family needs that are inevitable. I always caution aspiring doulas to place a premium on planning around this aspect of doula work. This is an adjustment for the entire family, one to be taken seriously and planned for. Although my postpartum doula work does not include the adrenaline-driven aspect of being "on call"—that feeling I experience when I work with birth doula clients—it remains spontaneous and unpredictable. After all, we don't know just when a baby will be born. Flexibility is a necessary part of doula work.

LAYING A FOUNDATION

Over the years, I have found that for things to go smoothly between home and work life, all family members must have realistic expectations of how life will be affected. Communication with clients, scheduling conflicts, and emotional preoccupation can ripple and affect the whole family. Experience has taught me that we can mitigate their impact with boundaries. I model the skill of protecting family time with my own behaviour. I do not make myself available to my clients round the clock. Although it may seem tempting and perhaps ideal to clients, this approach can lead to challenges at a brisk pace. My own experience early on taught me that doula burnout, blurred boundaries for the client (feeling encouraged to call you any time for any reason), and family resentment are all potential reasons for me to take a proactive approach when planning my transition from home to client and back to home.

YOU CAN'T TAKE IT WITH YOU

The next essential boundary is leaving my "coat" at the door. This means that as a doula, I leave my own life behind. My most immediate life—the sick child, the traffic—none of these are relevant to the support that I provide. Even more crucial to leave behind are the life experiences and opinions that form my core and identify me as a parent. This is where things get tricky. As a doula trainer, I explain that our experiences shape us; often, it's these experiences, positive or negative, that lead us to doula work. In mentoring doulas for over sixteen years, I have observed some doulas wanting to help others experience what they, the doulas, perceive to be triumphs—a natural birth, or breastfeeding, or a smooth transition. Others have been attracted to the work by a desire to protect women from something that they themselves experienced. Both are valid reasons to come to doula work. Neither reason can enter the client's home with the doula. When I work with families, I am there to help them meet their own objectives, not mine. Although this is sometimes an exercise in restraint on my part, it is a core of what I offer my clients—the trust that they can use the resources available to them to make the choices that feel right for their family.

My role is to come alongside my clients and to help them to determine their priorities and preferences and then to support them as they grow into their roles as confident parents. My clients will make their choices based on their own life experiences, just as I did. Much like the classic parent-child conundrum (i.e., telling your children, "Don't make the mistakes I made!"), it is impossible to expect other people to make decisions based on my own life experiences. This is a major cornerstone of my doula trainings. The doula who brings her story as a venue for bonding is missing an important element of the process of non-judgmental sharing. If I share my own story, I have set the bar either at what to do or what not to do. Both contain potential for damaging the doula-client relationship, as the mother now knows exactly what she is being measured against, even if she herself is the one doing the measuring. I have observed that experience in supporting families and providing evidence-based information is far more effective strategies for helping clients to navigate the many twists and turns that come with early parenting.

OUR BOUNDARIES DEFINE OUR PROFESSION

Once I leave my family and personal life at the door and am completely available to my clients, the next boundary is to stay within my role. The postpartum doula is an expert in being a generalist—neither diagnosing nor treating any condition. My job is to recognize when things are other than normal and know the steps to take when that happens. This boundary can be breached for a number of reasons: pride, enthusiasm, lack of alternatives and overconfidence, to name only a few. The doula who worries that she should be an expert in everything is more likely to make this mistake. Remember, no one is all-knowing. An honest answer is the best one. Experience has taught me that it is better to explain that I am not certain of an answer but know how to find it than it is to dole out misinformation.

A parallel risk can be the doula who feels overconfident in her knowledge base and considers it acceptable to provide support that would normally be provided by a specialist—perhaps with a breastfeeding challenge or in treating a client with essential oils. This situation offers space for error. Doulas are just that, doulas. We are not lactation specialists, clinical care providers, therapists, or bodyworkers. Taking on additional responsibilities dilutes our role and makes us less effective, even if we have training in those areas. As a doula, I focus on the essential skills: listening, guidance, and leading by following. These are made possible by my lack of additional responsibilities. Although some may worry that the generalist model of support may seem too broad or insufficient, I am certain that my ability to be present in any way necessary, without an agenda, is what allows me to serve families completely.

Occasionally, I have identified a challenge and referred my clients to specialists, but they were unwilling to reach out to them—perhaps because of financial reasons, the client feeling overwhelmed, or a difference of opinion. This placed me in an awkward situation since I had already identified the problem as being outside of my scope. It became especially important for me to establish and maintain my boundaries from the onset to avoid offering inappropriate support.

Many of us feel uncomfortable saying "no." I have learned that when I do so in a respectful and confident manner, things usually go quite well. It helps me to remember that the clarity of the role holds great merit. Certifying organizations, their standards and scopes provide support in this situation. So can doula mentors, trainers, and basic ethics. At each of my postpartum training workshops,

I offer these words of advice for new doulas: If someone asks you to do something that makes you uncomfortable, chances are that discomfort will only grow. Remain polite and respectful to your clients—as well as to yourself. Remember that your boundaries define both you and your profession.

OUTSIDE ROLES

Some individuals come to their doula work wearing multiple hats. It is not uncommon for a doula to present herself as a package—offering lactation support, or massage or childcare—in addition to doula support. Over the years, I have offered childbirth classes, pre or postnatal fitness coaching, and lactation support as well as birth and postpartum doula services. This is a natural result of expanding interests and the need for income. If these broad offerings are performed ethically and with consideration of boundaries, they can provide ideal opportunities for both parents and doula. Parents have the opportunity to experience a continuity of care that is missing in present-day culture. The same person who met them prenatally and attended their labour may now visit their home during the fourth trimester, for example, which fosters an ongoing relationship. As the doula, I benefit from opportunities to build strong relationships and to generate additional income. Where could this go wrong?

As I mentioned earlier, the doula role is a pure one—that of a generalist, without any other responsibilities. It is my very lack of a targeted agenda that allows me to remain open to following the parents wherever they need me most. The other more focused professions listed above require that an individual hone in on particular behaviours and situations, leaving less time to focus on other areas. This creates a risk of missing something important that isn't in our area of expertise. When working as a doula, I leave the "coat" of additional professions hanging next to my personal life at the door. If my clients and I decide together that they could benefit from additional services, I offer them referrals to visit other specialists. These are accompanied by a separate conversation about standards of practice, fees, and a separate contract. In this way, I remain mindful of the purity of my role so to ensure that parents are benefitting from actual doula services. Parents have the ability to choose a professional to fit their needs. Although an ongoing and transitioning relationship can be ideal, it needs to be done carefully. As their doula, I am now a trusted family confidante. It's important to me that I never leverage my position of trust to increase my working hours with a family. Offering my services as one of multiple options will help to take pressure off my clients.

Separate contracts help my clients and me. Oftentimes, more targeted roles such as lactation support and massage therapy come with a higher hourly income potential. If I offer my services through my regular shift, I will find myself paid at the rate of a postpartum doula—doing myself a financial disservice. In addition, clients might inaccurately incorporate this service into their expectation of doula services. Once again, as the person in the relationship with experience, I am the one to respectfully establish boundaries that will be beneficial for all.

CARING, NOT SHARING

Separating our own story from that of our clients' can be a challenging boundary for anyone. After all, I am immersed in the situation, and we, doula and client are experiencing an event together. I have my own important perspective of the situation, and my feelings are real and matter. I problem solve, resource, share sweat and tears at times. This story, however, belongs to the new parents. Their labour, their depression, their photographs, their challenges and successes—none of them are mine to share. Even with permission, it's wise for us as doulas to question our motivation when telling a client's story, anonymously or not. In a culture that thrives on public sharing, it seems natural to put our doula work out there, but we never know what others are thinking. We will never know what we might unintentionally post that could be hurtful or inappropriate, and our clients might never tell us. My personal priority, each time, is to keep my clients' stories and photos private.

There have been times when I have felt moved to share situations with peers for advice, or to process, or even to celebrate. These are appropriate if confidentiality is maintained. Names, identifying characteristics—neighborhoods, ethnicity and occupations, for example—should be avoided. The conversation relates only to my role, as that's what I need to process. This is what separates professionalism from gossip. Doula organizations place a premium on confidentiality, and all doulas must, as well. I strive to strike a balance between my need for support that can benefit me and my client while I remain mindful of the importance of confidentiality and of having a very basic respect for how people should treat one another.

DOULA EVOLUTION

With the name "doula" only having been adopted as an institution by Doulas of North America in 1992, we have been evolving as professionals for a relatively short time. As doulas gain name recognition and publicity, we experience shifts in who hires us and who chooses to work as a doula. With further changes in the economy, in issues pertaining to reproductive justice, and in the world at large, doulas will continue to adapt and their roles, evolve. Consider this: in 1992, there was limited use of the Internet, and it was only moderately popular by 2000. The economy was healthier then; more people were able to volunteer their services or work at a discount. Doulas today live in a different world. More and more women are drawn to doula work at a young age. College students consider it a viable profession, while their pregnant mothers likely did not know that doulas existed. People are coming to the field younger because they can—it now exists! They bring a new perspective, technological proficiency, and an internal belief in the legitimacy of the field that earlier doulas sometimes found challenging because they were blazing trails and defining the role with their very actions.

Newer generations of doulas are carving paths of their own. Social media, co-ops, online learning and marketing are changes that help the profession evolve to the next level and keep it current and appealing to upcoming generations. Newer doulas, entering a young but now-established field, usually have the expectation of a living wage—a fair expectation indeed. It can be fascinating to observe the clash of opinions on the topic of fees for doula services. As with most choices, they are based on a vast array of factors: finances, feminism, community, and even faith. Whichever choice the doula makes in terms of fees, boundaries will once again come into play. Setting fees and policies and clearly communicating these to clients is a must. Our role is inherently intimate and even the most business-minded doula may occasionally feel awkward when asking for payment at the end of a warm, oxytocin-induced session. In the early years of my own practice, even though I had great belief in what I was offering and confidence in the fees that I was setting, I found the actual conversations and policies regarding the business end of my work to be stressful and awkward. This is another area where both boundaries and experience make all the difference. Planning ahead and having established procedures and protocols, all accessible in writing, help to keep this aspect of doula work running smoothly.

Fortunately, just as there is a doula match out there for every woman who wants one, there is an approach and an organization for every doula. Rather than debating a particular philosophy, doulas can hopefully recognize that the non-judgmental approach that defines our role must extend to peers. There is room for diversity in the doula world. As with our clients, we can have opinions and preferences and advocate for those on a macro-level and maintain the healthy and respectful boundary of embracing difference and diversity when interacting with doulas we meet who approach things differently.

SEPARATING OURSELVES FROM OUR CLIENTS

Yet another essential priority is separating my clients' experiences from my own. Just as I can't bring my own experiences and project them onto my client, I shouldn't absorb hers. Boundaries must exist in both directions. Doula work cannot be based on outcomes. As a doula, I am not successful if my client meets certain criteria, such as breastfeeding success. Nor do my client's perceived challenges belong to me. My success is in maintaining my role: working alongside the parents and meeting them where they are. If a doula comes alongside her clients with an open and accepting heart, offers options and nurturing support, and makes herself unnecessary in the process, she is successful. Our criterion for success ends where it begins—with our roles and boundaries.

III.
Doulas and Institutions

11.
Being a Doula When Birth Choice is Limited

Supporting Birthing Mothers
in a Mexican Hospital

VANIA SMITH-OKA

T HE BIRTHING SYSTEM FOR LOW-INCOME WOMEN in many Mexican public hospitals is less than ideal. Most hospitals are underfunded, understaffed, and overstrained (Gómez-Dantés et al. S227; Walker et al. 19). Emphasis is placed on moving women in labour as rapidly as possible through the system, with little regard for their welfare. Hospital policies separate labouring women from their sources of support from the moment that the women enter the labour and delivery ward. What little support that they do receive comes from overworked physicians and nurses, who are not trained to alleviate women's fears and concerns about birth. Women thus give birth alone, vulnerable, and frightened.

The aim of my larger ethnographic research was to investigate the culture of a labour ward, particularly regarding risk, medical space, and birth outcomes. I never expected to be drawn into the emotional and physical needs of the patients in such a fundamental way. I became an unexpected doula in the patients' labours, whereby I provided emotional support, breathing advice, and backrubs. Based on ethnographic research at a maternity ward in a public hospital in the city of Puebla, Mexico, I address the important perspective that participating as a doula provides. I share women's stories of despair and hope, fear and vulnerability, horror and joy to raise critical questions about provider-patient interactions and humanized forms of birth. The question that specifically drives this article is, what sort of role can doulas play in contexts where the patients have little choice over their own birth experiences? Can doulas successfully support women in these situations?

Social support is necessary for birthing women (Campero et al. 401; Morton 88; Hodnett et al. 21; Gilliland 525; Hunter 316; Morton and Clift 37; Shlafer et al. 2). Much of the research on this issue emphasizes that women who receive support during labour or birth have better physical and emotional outcomes than women who do not receive this support. Conversely, women who lack social support are more likely to have complications during their pregnancy (Deitrick and Draves 397). Social support can be defined as the transfer of knowledge, advice, or information that makes people feel that they are engaged in a broader connection and interaction with others. Zimet et al. (31) describe the complexities of social support: its content (verbal, emotional, etc.), direction (reciprocal, unidirectional), or whether it is direct support or serves as a buffering agent. Rosen (24) lists the components of social support during labour: emotional (reassurance, praise, continuous presence), physical (comfort measures), and informational (information about what is happening and advice about how to cope). She also adds the need for advocacy (i.e., respecting a woman's decisions and helping to communicate them to clinicians). Deitrick and Draves (398) attribute emotional ties to social support and add that a person's well-being is related to social support.

Scholars have robustly shown that the presence of a doula during birth supports labouring women in multiple ways, from reducing the use of epidurals (Gordon et al. 424) and Caesarean sections (Campero et al. 321; Kozhimannil et al. e3) to increasing satisfaction with the overall birth experience (Hodnett et al. 9). Gilliland (525) states that support by doulas has been one of the most important innovations in birth care: not only does doula care have many positive effects, but it most importantly has no known negative effects on the mother or baby. She adds that doula care overlaps only slightly with the care provided by nurses; the majority of doula care (mirroring, reinforcing, debriefing, etc.) is not provided by any other caregiver. In addition, doulas provide continuity of care that is so necessary for labouring women. Thus doula care is much more complex than previously thought. Hunter (320) proposes that doulas create and hold an intimate space, tangible or ethereal, so that a patient may feel protected and safe. Doulas are not solely a support or cost-effective option (Kozhimannil et al. e8); they also fill important gaps in childbirth care not provided by others. Recent work by Shlafer (2) among incarcerated pregnant women shows that the presence of doulas dramatically improves the birth experience and outcome. Doulas in these prisons also emotionally support the women after they are separated from their newborn infants. They are thus integral to the women's well-being.

Most research on doulas has taken place in the global North (Gordon et al. 423; Morton 53; Fisher et al. 64; Gilliland 525; Hunter 315; Morton and Clift 98). These researchers explore issues such as the effect of doulas on birth outcomes, women's personal experiences with doulas, or the role of doulas in empowering women during birth. Whether by a partner, family, or other support person, such as a doula, social support has increasingly become routine in hospital births in these countries. Only a few projects, however, explore the presence of doulas or other forms of social support in global South countries, such as Campero et al.'s (395) work in Mexico, Sosa et al.'s (587) study in Guatemala, Alexander et al.'s (4) work in Ghana, or Oboro et al.'s (56) and Morhason-Bello et al.'s (554) research in Nigeria, to name a few. As Oboro et al. point out, the presence of any form of social support (mother, partner, doula) in many non-industrialized countries is not routine practice. Indeed, in many of these countries, support companions are often denied access to labouring women. Additionally, within many hospital contexts—whether in the global North or South—there is little choice offered to the patients about what their birth should entail. This is a significant gap as it speaks to the inconsistencies in birth systems: global South countries are striving to improve maternal health care while simultaneously ignoring support systems that contribute to the better health care statistics in the global North.

RESEARCHING BIRTH IN MEXICO

This research began with a question, how do large urban public hospitals manage patients' labours and births, considering the structural issues of space, low resources, and overworked staff? I was interested in exploring how resources were used in the hospital, how patients viewed their birth experiences, and whether midwives played any role in their prenatal care. As is the case with most ethnography, the research changed as I arrived at the field site and witnessed the birth experiences of the patients at this hospital in the city of Puebla.

Puebla is a city of approximately 1.5 million people in central Mexico (INEGI). A relatively wealthy city, known for its universities, museums, and car industry (both Volkswagen and Audi have large assembly plants), it also has tremendous disparities between the rich and poor (INEGI). The city is the economic and political powerhouse of the state of Puebla; the rural and hinterland regions of the state are very marginalized. Such disparity means that the state has some of the worst statistics in the country for educational attainment, maternal mortality, and neonatal birth weight, to name only a few categories (INEGI). In the city of Puebla, approximately 650 thousand people have no access to formal health care (CEIGEP). Just over 100 000 families are enrolled in Seguro Popular (INEGI).[1] The city has 111 medical centers—most of which are small clinics staffed by fewer than five clinicians. In 2012, the ratio of medical personnel in public hospitals/clinics was 2.99 for every 1,000 people (CEIGEP). Nationally, the state of Puebla has the sixth highest rate of low-weight births (8.5 percent); it also has one of the highest rates of home births in the nation (12.2 percent). Physicians attend almost 80 percent of the clinical births. Nurses attend to the rest (CEIGEP).

To address the population's health issues, several large public hospitals have been built over the last decade, including Hospital Público (a pseudonym), where my research took place. Hospital Público attends to approximately 9,000 births a year (around 850 a month). In 2009, it had 142 physicians (from interns to full-time) and 290 nurses on staff. In 2011, it had 65 registered beds and 150 unregistered ones (gurneys, labour beds, and those in the labour and delivery ward). Other numbers—which have remained relatively constant over the years and notably affect quality of care—are significant in this hospital: its daily capacity (140 percent),[2] its Caesarean section rate (45 percent), and its rate of adolescent birth, under 18 years of age (25 percent). These numbers are part of the underlying structure that shapes the complicated birth process at this hospital.

My data is based on research carried out during 2008 and 2011, during which I undertook over 120 hours of participant observation. Over the course of a variety of interviews with clinicians and patients (ranging from sit down interviews to casual chats in the wards), I spoke with 30 physicians, 9 nurses, and 71 female patients. Most of the patients (70 percent) were first-time mothers. Additionally, in 2011, I interviewed 10 midwives who were being professionalized at the hospital. I also participated as a doula in the birth of ten women. After their birth, we spoke in depth about their sense of empowerment and satisfaction with their birth.

BIRTH AT THE HOSPITAL

Typewriters always remind me of the birthing ward at Hospital Público. This outdated technology was the mainstay of recordkeeping. Physicians dragged heavy typewriters from one patient to another as they painstakingly typed out patients' responses to structured questions about their age, address, and number of pregnancies. The clickety-clack of typing was interspersed with moans and cries from the many patients in labour in the ward. Some days the ward was almost empty, with only one or two patients labouring alone in a labour cubicle. Other days, the ward resembled a disaster zone, with patients on gurneys lined up along all available walls in various stages of labour or postpartum, attended to by harried and overworked nurses and physicians.

Birth in this hospital is designed around a technocratic model (Davis-Floyd 56). Similar to what Campero et al. (396) show in their work on social support in hospital childbirth in Mexico, Hospital Público's policy does not allow partners, mothers, or other forms of support to accompany the patient into the labour-delivery ward. Patients were thus separated from anyone who knew them. They were moved through the system, from intake to recovery, based on specific hospital measures. When patients entered the birthing ward at the discretion of the intake physician, they were placed on a gurney in a labour cubicle—narrow Plexiglas spaces slightly wider than a gurney. There, they were attached to an intravenous drip of fluids and Pitocin. They were expected to lie down during the duration of the labour. Hospital policy dictated that patients could not consume anything (neither food nor water) during labour and delivery. Pain medication was unavailable, the hospital's short supply reserved for Caesarean sections. During this time, patients were repeatedly examined for the ten centimeter cervical dilation necessary for transfer to the next stage (Smith-Oka 596 *Managing Labor*). Their only contact with other people during labour was through the vaginal examinations, the intake questions, and the occasional social worker or psychology student asking questions about birth control and family planning. Patients thus laboured alone, tethered, vulnerable, and unable to make any decisions about their birth.

AN UNEXPECTED DOULA

My first foray into this research was in 2008. I had no first-hand experience with the process of medicalized hospital birth, and even less with how to support birthing women. I was introduced to the birthing system at this hospital in Mexico during Estefanía's delivery.[3] She was a young, sixteen-year-old first-time mother who was utterly fearful and confused about birth. She had no idea what was going on as she lay on a birthing table in the middle of the delivery room, surrounded by almost a dozen dispassionate clinicians. Her entire body language—tense, looking around with wide eyes, asking repeatedly if the baby was out—revealed her fear and vulnerability. Yet no one helped her or spoke to her except to scold. I had entered the room with one of the young female residents, originally planning to simply keep out of the way and observe births. But Estefanía's pleas drew me to her, and I found myself holding her hand, stroking her hair, and mumbling how she was doing fine and the baby would be out soon. I felt incompetent and unskilled. This feeling was compounded by the fact that, despite all of Estefanía's efforts, her birth was ultimately a Caesarean section.

This experience as a doula was followed in rapid succession by several other women's births, some vaginal and some Caesarean. Regardless of what sort of birth they had, each of these women's experiences was marked by a significant lack of power and control over their bodies, their decisions, and their births.

Isabel's birth exemplifies many of these issues—lack of power, the fear, and my unexpected role as a doula. Isabel was a young, married, nineteen-year-old woman, pregnant with her first child. We met while she was on a labour gurney, attached to a bag dripping Pitocin. Lying on her back, she was experiencing very strong contractions. I rubbed her back and helped her to shift position onto her side, where she clung to the railing. During each contraction, I would press her lower back, which seemed to alleviate her pain. She said she felt both hot and sleepy.

After some, time she felt her contractions come faster and said she wanted to push, so I called Dr. B., a young male resident with a friendly open manner. He told her she was nine centimeters dilated. Her Pitocin was increased to about one drip every two seconds, augmenting her contractions significantly. Isabel contorted on the bed with each contraction, clutching my hand, and crying in pain. Soon, another physician, Dr. T., a handsome and flirtatious man, came to check her. He determined that she had to have an emergency Caesarean section because the fetal heart rate was distressed. Isabel looked frightened; she turned to me and asked if I would be allowed to go in with her. Tears came to my eyes at her plaintive question.

Isabel held my hand tightly while she was prepped for the surgery. After she was wheeled into one of the delivery rooms, she was told to move from her gurney to the operating table on her own. She laboriously shuffled across. No one helped her. Dr. G., a female anesthesiologist, prepped her for an epidural and told her to turn onto her side. Isabel, exhausted and confused, struggled to roll onto the correct position. I was unable to support her because I would have been in the way of all the medical preparation. I finally found a small spot by Dr. G., and held Isabel's hand, trying to comfort her. She squeezed my hand in return.

Telling her to bend her legs, clinicians then rolled Isabel onto her back. They put povidone iodine across her abdomen and vagina as well as poured a blood-red liquid on her abdomen from a metal jar, gruesomely presaging her abdominal surgery. Her arms were placed at right angles to her body, loosely tied with bandages to wooden boards placed under her mattress. Blue sterile sheets were placed across her body, legs, and in front of her face. Two surgeons—Dr. B. and Dr. L. (a female second-year resident)—scrubbed up and were outfitted with surgery garb. I stayed at Isabel's head but could no longer hold her hand. There was a strong sense of urgency among the clinicians. The surgeons did not know her name and could not find her chart. I helped with as many details as I could, including her name, age, and pregnancy status. Soon afterwards, the surgery began. Her baby girl was born a few minutes later and was taken by the neonatologist to clean and measure. I stroked Isabel's hair and told her she had a lovely girl. Her happy smile, filtered through an epidural haze, was followed by an exhausted sleep.

Victoria's case, occurring in 2011, was different from both Estefanía's and Isabel's. She was not a first-time mother, having given birth to two children more than nine years before. These births had been at home with a midwife, and thus she felt her hospital birth was particularly jarring. I was also different that year, as I had trained as a doula in a course in 2008 (though never certified) and felt more competent to support women emotionally and physically.

Victoria had gone to the hospital unwillingly, solely as a re-quirement of her enrollment in Seguro Popular. During labour, she experienced an agonizing set of vaginal examinations designed to open up her cervix and speed up birth[4] from Dr. R. I spent a long time with her during active labour, holding her hand, rub-bing her back as needed, trying to comfort her. She softly whis-pered, "That doctor hurts me a lot. I am very afraid." Once she had dilated to ten centimeters, she was wheeled into a delivery room. As with Isabel above, Victoria had to shuffle across from her gurney to the delivery table on her own. She searched for my hand and begged me not to leave her. I was given the bag of fluids to hang up, as I was closest to the IV stand. Her birth was both aggressive and rapid. She barely had to push, as Dr. R. reached his hand into her vagina and drew the baby out manually. Victoria screamed out in pain and looked up at me with terrified eyes, begging, "Don't leave me, don't leave me." Holding her hand, I urged her to concentrate on my face and not think of the pain. Her baby girl was born barely ten minutes later and was taken by the neonatologists to clean and measure. I stayed with Victoria until she was transferred to the immediate postpartum room, where I helped her to latch her baby onto her breast and commence feeding.

A few days postpartum, I visited her at home, where she spoke about her fears and concerns with her birth. Part of our conversation is below:

> Victoria: "You don't know the pleasure it was to have you there at the birth with me. I was very afraid, as I had never given birth in the hospital and the doctor was hurting me.... It felt horrible how he hurt me. Now I can feel like some cramps on side of my [female] part."

> Vania: "The thing is that the doctor opened up your cervix forcefully (*a la fuerza*). He put in his hand ... and opened up the neck of the uterus."

> Victoria: "It felt horrible. A terrible pain. I could feel how he pulled and I felt as if he removed something.... Are all of [the doctors] like that there?"

> Vania: "No, he likes to do it that way, but there are all kinds at the hospital."

> Victoria: "I was so afraid. And you came up to me and I felt so much happiness. I tell my husband that you were my salvation, my guardian angel. And even though the doctor was polite, he hurt me a lot.... And there were so many people there! I am not used to that, as I gave birth to my other children here [at home]."

Victoria's words were illustrative of several other female patients' experiences at the hospital. Her feelings of fear, helplessness, and confusion were shared by others. What was different from other women was the fact that she had had prior birth experiences, which she compared favorably to this hospital birth. My presence as a doula and the social support that I provided allowed Victoria to focus her emotions and her body to overcome the physician-caused fear and pain.

VOICES OF MIDWIVES

During 2011, there was a group of over thirty female (and one male) midwives who were being professionalized by the hospital. They ranged from traditional birth attendants, to lay midwives who had learned their techniques over years, to nurses who were allowed to attend births in private/public clinics. This fascinating group of practitioners was enrolled in a three-month course that included theory and practical observation of labour and birth. The theory classes were dry Power Point-based presentations imparted by first year medical students or seasoned nurses. The practical observation consisted of a once-a-week admittance in small groups into the labour ward. In the words of the nurse in charge of the class, "You will realize how things are in there.... You will [be allowed] into the operating room. You will see how they do cesareans and how they take the baby out."

In the labour ward, the midwives were explicitly told that their role was to observe, not to intervene. They were there to learn, not to criticize. The midwives for the most part followed these rules. They would go up to women in labour, and ask how they were doing, hold their hands, or help them to breathe. Many times, they would rest against the walls of the ward and would chat among themselves about their practices, their observations, or their critiques. One young midwife, who proudly told us that she had just received her nursing degree that week, spent a long time with one anxious labouring mother, talking with her and gently stroking her forehead. She spent over an hour with her, after which the mother said, "I can feel how my body relaxes." Some of the patients felt better with our presence, as one patient expressed after I massaged her, "I feel more relaxed when you touch me."

The midwives voiced a lot of critique and concerns about the treatment of the patients. Emilia, who had worked as a nurse for twenty-three years, whispered to me as she saw a male physician carry out a vaginal exam with no lubrication, "Look at that. He does not tell her, 'Look, ma'am I'm going to examine you' nor does he put on lubricant. Very bad!" Later, as we left the hospital together, she voiced even more scathing critique, "The treatment here is very poor. It's because it is a public hospital. That would never happen at a private [one]."

FEELING IMPOTENT: LIMITS OF CHOICE

This paper is driven by the question of what sort of role doulas can play in contexts where the patients have no choice over their own birth experiences. I address the issue of provider-patient interactions, in particular aspects of humanized forms of birth.

Estefanía's, Isabel's, and Victoria's births exemplify many of the other births that I witnessed during my research at the hospital. These first-hand accounts were also observed by other researchers in the hospital as well as by the midwives. One midwife, Almudena, with many years of experience in home births, said to me, "But the patient is a human being like any other, no? ... They are supposedly attending a human being, not at animal. Even the cows have their [birth] time, right?"[5] Her words resonate with Victoria's fears and lack of control over her birth experience, focusing on one of the core issues present in the births at this hospital: the absence of humanized birth.

Campero et al. (396) emphasize patient concerns with giving birth alone, and the anxiety this produces. Despite important research demonstrating that anxiety, fear, and stress in childbirth can have consequences for the birth process, women's health, and birth outcomes (Fisher et al. 65), most hospitals in Mexico as yet do not recognize the importance of social support. Campero et al. (396) refer to this sort of birth experience as "mechanical and intimidating." All the patients whom I mentioned were anxious. In Isabel's case, her fear and anxiety, coupled with the excessive use of Pitocin, likely sent her body into distress, which resulted in a Caesarean section.

My data shows that the birth experience was certainly intimidating for the patients. None of them was guided through the birth process by clinicians. There were almost no forms of social support (verbal, emotional, or physical) and none involving psycho-social comfort (Deitrick and Draves 403). Few times did they receive explanations of what was happening or why. Patients frequently heard the refrain of "cooperate, help the doctors, and all will be fine" during their birth. Patients tended to interpret this refrain as a threat: if they did not cooperate there would be consequences. They expressed significant fear, nervousness, or concern about their birth experiences.

The birth process was mechanical for the patients—unthinking, unfeeling, unmoving. They were subject to the hospital's bureaucratic rules and procedures with no option but to comply. But this process was also mechanical for the clinicians. To address the high number of patients, physicians had designed a shorthand set of indicators (cervical dilation, rate of contractions, time spent in the labour cubicle) to move women through the birth process as rapidly and seamlessly as possible. Not only did clinicians have no time to deal with each patient individually, they were not trained to expect uncomplicated births or those that entailed a more humanized and supportive approach. As voiced by Dr. R, who attended Victoria's birth, "It is better to have ten minutes of pain than two to three hours of slow contractions" adding that if the baby took too long and patients were allowed to labour naturally, then the baby could asphyxiate. So he would rather have fast labours and deliveries. The physician's job was thus akin to that of a traffic cop: directing and dictating the bodies of their innumerable patients to prevent any traffic jams. As Walker et al. (26) state, there is significant room for including other forms of birth attendants into the birth system in Mexico. Such an addition would serve the important functions of improving health care for labouring women as well as alleviate the pressures placed on physicians by sharing the workload and workspace with multiple birth specialists.

A particular issue that was very present in my research was the limits of choice. At no point in their labours were patients consulted about options and possibilities. Their bodies were moved, cut, or opened at the behest of others. The patients thus had a marked lack of control. They had no voice in any part of their labour and birth, whether about labour position, the presence of oxytocin or even in the type of birth that they ultimately had.

The patients in my study differed greatly from those in other studies about doulas. Although Gordon et al. (425) or Campero et al. (401) state that women supported by doulas have much better outcomes, were more likely to express that they had had a good birth experience, coped well with labour, and considered their body's strength and abilities in a positive way, this was not necessarily the case with the patients in my study. Perhaps this can be attributed to a lack in my own doulaing abilities or those of the midwives. I would, however, suggest that the primarily reason for the patients' problematic birth outcomes is the larger institutional constrains embedded within birth systems in public hospitals in Mexico. Although the labouring women might have appreciated my presence or that of the midwives—as calming, supportive, caring, allowing them to relax—it had little influence on their outcome, the type of birth that they experienced, or even their level of satisfaction.

Because of the training physicians received, their high number of patients, and their need to move them through the birth unit, they were unable to see a doula as anything but another body, another medical practitioner. They were not trained to understand the role of doulas, or the possible benefits that they could provide. Because doulas are considered a non-entity in this setting, neither the patients nor the midwives nor I had any power to advocate. This powerlessness was captured by one of the midwives who stated after spending time in the labour ward, "You feel so impotent [there]."

Returning to the types of social support for women in labour (emotional, physical, informational, advocacy, and psycho-social comfort) that I described above, it is evident that in situations where patients have little control or power, doulas can have a role, although different from the one available in other contexts. Some of these forms of support (emotional, informational) can continue to be present. The midwives and I were all able to provide reassurance and praise as emotional support to the patients, and we were able to explain to them what certain procedures consisted of. Others forms (physical, psycho-social) can be present in a reduced manner: the patients could receive backrubs or other gentle forms of physical comfort, but they would not be able to get off the labour gurney and walk around.

I argue that advocacy, however, is almost impossible in these situations as physicians are the primary decision makers, and doulas (whether I as researcher or the midwives as students) are only granted access at a physician's discretion. In a hierarchical system such as this, where decision makers were full-time physicians or hospital administrators, there was no scope for advocacy or for a gentler form of birth.

LAST THOUGHTS

This article has been an analysis of whether doulas can serve any role in contexts with little birth choice. Based on evidence gathered from patients, clinicians, and midwives, I have provided a lens through which this issue can be addressed. While my findings are disheartening, they nevertheless show that doulas cannot provide the sort of support to patients labouring in contexts of little choice that they would like to. The role of doulas in these contexts seems to be of micro-support: providing a small intimate space of relaxation (Hunter 320) and allowing the patient to feel cared for and supported in a chaotic birth environment. Shlafer et al.'s work among doulas attending to imprisoned women is an intriguing framework of practices outside of the normal parameters of birth attendance. As they emphasize, in contexts where institutional restrictions can constrain the usual doula-client relationship, doulas have to become more adept at creating a space of emotional support for such patients. A greater amount of research is needed on this issue of doulaing within institutional constraints to delve deeper into additional effects doulas can have on patient welfare and outcome.

ENDNOTES

[1]Launched in 2003, Seguro Popular is aimed at populations previously uninsured or who lacked access to health care. It is designed to help low-income families to cover health-related needs. One of its primary goals is to reduce the prevalence of catastrophic health expenditures (Knaul et al. 2).

[2]A well-running hospital should be at about 80 percent.

[3]I have elaborated on her birth story in other articles (Smith-Oka *Bodies of Risk* 2279). In these works, I discuss ideas of risk, adolescence, and bad motherhood, and the ways that young mothers are classified as problem mothers and are treated accordingly by the clinicians.

[4]As with Estefanía, I have elaborated on Victoria's birth in other articles (Smith-Oka *Managing Labor* 596). In this work, I specifically address the routinizing of cervical exams and the problems that this creates for women and the birth system in general.

[5]I elaborate on some of the concerns of midwives in other articles (Smith-Oka *Managing Labor* 601).

WORKS CITED

Alexander, Amir, et al. "Social Support During Delivery in Rural Central Ghana: A Mixed Methods Study of Women's Preferences for and Against Inclusion of a Lay Companion in the Delivery Room." *Journal of Biosocial Science* 46.5 (2014): 669-685. Print.

Campero, Lourdes, et al. "'Alone, I Wouldn't Have Known What to Do': A QualitativeStudy on Social Support During Labor and Delivery in Mexico." *Social Science & Medicine* 41.3 (1998): 395-403. Print.

Campero, Lourdes, et al. "Support from a Prenatal Instructor During Childbirth Is Associated with Reduced Rates of Caesarean Section in a Mexican Study." *Midwifery* 20.4 (2004): 312-323. Print.

Comité Estatal de Información Estadística y Geográfica del Estado de Puebla (CEIGEP). *Comité Estatal de Información Estadística y Geográfica del Estado de Puebla.* CEIGEP, 2012. Web. 26 Aug. 2014.

Davis-Floyd, R. "The Technocratic, Humanistic, and Holistic Paradigms of Childbirth." *International Journal of Gynecology and Obstetrics* 75.1 (2001): S5-S23. Print.

Deitrick, Lynn M., and Patrick R. Draves. "Attitudes towards Doula Support during Pregnancy by Clients, Doulas, and Labor-and-Delivery Nurses: A Case Study from Tampa, Florida." *Human Organization* 67.4 (2008): 397-406. Print.

Fisher, Colleen, Yvonne Hauck, and Jenny Fenwick. "How Social

Context Impacts on Women's Fears of Childbirth: A Western Australian Example." *Social Science and Medicine* 63.1 (2006): 64-75. Print.

Gilliland, Amy L. "After Praise and Encouragement: Emotional Support Strategies Used by Birth Doulas in the USA and Canada." *Midwifery* 27.4 (2011): 525-531. Print.

Gómez-Dantés, Octavio, et al. "Sistema de Salud de México." *Salud Pública de México* 53.2 (2011): S220-S232. Print.

Gordon, Nancy P., et al. "Effects of Providing Hospital-Based Doulas in Health Maintenance Organization Hospitals." *Obstetrics & Gynecology* 93.3 (1999): 422-426. Print.

Hodnett, E.D., et al. "Continuous Support for Women During Childbirth (Review)." *Cochrane Database of Systematic Reviews* 3 (2007): 1-68. Print.

Hunter, Cheryl. "Intimate Space within Institutionalized Birth: Women's Experiences Birthing with Doulas." *Anthropology & Medicine* 19.3 (2012): 315-326. Print.

Instituto Nacional de Estadística y Geografía Instituto (INEGI). *Nacional de Estadística y Geografía.* INEGI, n.d. Web. 20 August 2014.

Knaul, Felicia M., et al. "The Quest for Universal Health Coverage: Achieving Social Protection for All in Mexico." *The Lancet* 380.9849 (2012): 1259-1279. Print.

Kozhimannil, Katy B., et al. "Doula Care, Birth Outcomes and Costs Among Medicaid Beneficiaries." *American Journal of Public Health* 103.4 (2013): e113-e121. Print.

Morton, Christine. *Doula Care: The (Re)-Emergence of Woman-Supported Childbirth in the United States.* Diss. UCLA, 2002. Ann Arbor: ProQuest UMI, 2002. Print.

Morton, Christine H., and Elayne Clift. *Birth Ambassadors: Doulas and the Re-emergence of Woman-Supported Birth in America.* Amarillo, TX: Praeclarus Press, 2014. Print.

Morhason-Bello, I. O., et al. "Attitude and Preferences of Nigerian Antenatal Women to Social Support During Labour." *Journal of Biosocial Science* 40.4 (2008): 553-562. Print.

Oboro, Victor O., et al. "Attitudes of Nigerian Women toward the Presence of Their Husband or Partner as a Support Person During Labor." *International Journal of Gynecology and Ob-*

stetrics 112.1 (2011): 56-58. Print.

Shlafer, Rebecca J., et al. "Doulas' Perspectives about Providing Support to Incarcerated Women: A Feasibility Study." *Public Health Nursing* 32.4 (2015): 316-326. Print.

Smith-Oka, Vania. "Bodies of Risk: Constructing Motherhood in a Mexican Public Hospital." *Social Science & Medicine* 75 (2012): 2275-2282. Print.

Smith-Oka, Vania. "Managing Labor and Delivery among Impoverished Populations in Mexico: Cervical Examinations as Bureaucratic Practice." *American Anthropologist* 115.4 (2013): 595-607. Print.

Sosa, Roberto, et al. "The Effect of a Supportive Companion on Perinatal Problems, Length of Labor, and Mother-Infant Interaction." *The New England Journal of Medicine* 303.11 (1980): 597-600. Print.

Walker, Dilys, et al. "Skilled Birth Attendants in Mexico: How Does Care During Normal Birth by General Physicians, Obstetric Nurses, and Professional Midwives Compare with World Health Organization Evidence-Based Practice Guidelines?" *Journal of Midwifery & Women's Health* 57.1 (2012): 18-27. Print.

Zimet, Gregory D., et al. "The Multidimensional Scale of Perceived Social Support." *Journal of Personality Assessment* 52.1 (1988): 30-41. Print.

12.
Cultivating Collaborative Relationships in the Provision of Labour Support

Doulas and Labour and Delivery Nurses

CHRISTINE MORTON, MARLA SEACRIST, JENNIFER TORRES, AND NICOLE HEIDBREDER

C HILDBIRTH LABOUR IS AN EMBODIED ACTIVITY where labour support has been shown to be an important source of emotional and physical comfort for women during childbirth (Hodnett, Gates, Hofmeyr, and Sakala). But who can best provide labour support, and what it entails, has yet to be clearly defined in the literature. Continuous support has been shown to improve maternal outcomes, and some studies report that labour support can be provided by untrained or trained women, relatives, nurses, and midwives (Barrett and Stark 13; Morton and Clift 171; Rosen 25).

There have been several attempts to define the content and scope of supportive care in labour. Some describe labour support as human presence and acceptance, which includes emotional support, physical support, information and advice, advocacy, and caregiver support (Rosen 24); others emphasize the components of physical and psychosocial comfort (Deitrick and Draves 401); and some include emotional support, physical comfort, instructional, and advocacy (Bianchi and Adams 25).

However labour support is defined, anthropological data suggests that in all but one of 128 cultures studied worldwide, a family member or friend remains with a woman throughout labour and birth (Trevathan 135). Female support was a key feature of U.S. births through the turn of the twentieth century when most American women gave birth at home, attended to by their close female relatives and friends who brought with them generations' worth of everyday knowledge and experience (Bogdan 92; Leavitt 87).

However, the rapid shift in birth location from home to hospital in the 1940s and 1950s dramatically altered the preeminent role of women's social networks, leaving women with only the labour and delivery nurse for supportive care (Morton and Clift 61). In the current U.S. context, a family or friend acting as a support person, a labour and delivery nurse, or increasingly, a doula, provides most labour-support activities.

Emerging as a specific labour-support role in U.S. maternity care over the past thirty-five years, doulas now attend approximately five to six percent of all births in the United States (Declercq, Sakala, Corry, Applebaum, and Herrlich 16; Morton and Clift 32). Researchers have variously articulated the doula role to include five aspects—labour-support skills, guidance and encouragement, assistance in care gaps, building team relationships, and encouraging communication between patient and caregivers (Gilliland "Beyond Holding Hands" 763)—or four elements: emotional support, physical comfort, instructional, and advocacy (Bianchi and Adams 25).

The medical maternity system in the U.S. and Canada often does not provide for one-to-one care (Gilliland "After Praise and Encouragement" 529), and nurses are hindered in providing labour support by several separate but interconnected factors, including unit staffing patterns affecting nurse-patient ratios, hospital policies, documentation responsibilities as well as a subculture that devalues emotional or hands-on supportive care (Barrett and Stark 14; Rosen 28).

Researchers have argued that doulas emerged in the U.S. context in part as a response to medicalized care and the increasing technological and documentation tasks required of labour and delivery nurses (Morton and Clift 223). The doula role does not include clinical tasks or responsibilities, yet most doulas accomplish their care in a highly medicalized institutional context—the hospital.

For doulas, providing labour support in a hospital setting means that they must carefully navigate and negotiate boundaries regarding their scope with maternity clinicians also present (Torres 924). The clinician most likely to have overlapping roles with a doula is the labour and delivery nurse.

BOUNDARIES AND BODIES:
DOULAS AND NURSES' ROLES IN THE LABOUR ROOM

Doulas care for a birthing woman through the use of emotional and physical comfort practices, and stay vigilant to signs of distress or stress in her body throughout the entire course of labour. Similarly, the nurses' attention is focused on the birthing woman's emotional and physical distress, but nurses must also assess fetal well-being and respond to fetal compromise, whether intrauterine or at birth. The nurses' focus, then, is divided between labouring women and their babies. Nurses monitor labouring women by checking their vital signs, cervical change, assessments of pain, and simultaneously conduct ongoing assessment of fetal and newborn status.

Doulas are typically present with women throughout the entire labour and, by virtue of this continuous presence, can feel a sense of "ownership" over birthing women's bodies and labour experience. Doulas, however, are not privy to fetal health and well-being. Although not present throughout the entire labour, nurses have access to information about the woman, her fetus, and the birthing context that doulas are unlikely to access. Nurses may view the medical record, an external account of women's experience, and may also be more informed about the obstetric provider's orders and preferences for labour management as well as hospital policies that constrain and facilitate women's labour experience.

Most doulas are hired directly by pregnant women and are primarily accountable to their clients. Independently hired doulas may also be accountable to all other doulas, since any one doula's behavior may influence clinicians' views on all doulas. Nurses are accountable to birthing women as patients in a context that requires them to be accountable to institutional policies and liabilities for poor outcomes. Nurses are assigned birthing women as patients in an institution that demands much more of them, as employees, than ensuring that any particular woman feels supported and cared for. These additional demands on nurses' time and attention include monitoring fetal well-being, juggling multiple patient loads, working under constant threat of liability, responsibility to adhere to institutional policies, implementing orders from providers, all while attending to the clinical and emotional needs of laboring women. In this chapter, we present data from two studies to high-light particular boundary challenges that can arise between doulas and nurses and how they view each other's role, and to suggest ways for collaborative care of birthing women.

METHODS

Data for this chapter are drawn from two studies. The first set of data, part of a larger qualitative study, comes from interviews with eighteen DONA International doulas and four labour and delivery nurses conducted between January 2011 and December 2012 in the Midwest region of the United States. Participants were assigned pseudonyms. Doulas were recruited through DONA International's website, www.dona.org, and nurses were recruited through snowball sampling. The second set of data comes from the *Maternity Support Survey (MSS)*, an online survey of doulas, childbirth educators, and labour and delivery nurses in the U.S. and Canada conducted from November 2012 through March 2013 using Survey Monkey. Approximately 2,600 respondents were recruited through membership organizations, social media, and snowball sampling.

FINDINGS: HOW DOULAS AND NURSES VIEW EACH OTHER

We asked doula and nurse respondents in the *Maternity Support Survey* how they viewed each other (Figure one). Just under half (46 percent) of the labour nurses in the *Maternity Support Survey* agreed with the statement, "Doulas are collaborative team members." As well, less than half of the nurses agreed that doula presence in labour enhances communication around women's birth experiences (43 percent). The item with the strongest level of agreement was that doulas enhance the women's birth experience (63 percent), underscoring nurses' recognition of the emotional benefits of labour support. Just one quarter of nurses agreed that "Doulas interfere with the nurse-doula relationship" and 19 percent agreed that doulas interfere with nurses' ability to provide care to a labouring woman. About 30 to 35 percent of nurses had no opinion on these issues, perhaps reflecting their lack of experience

Figure One: How Doulas and Nurses View Each Other (N=896 Nurses; N=1269 Doulas), *Maternity Support Survey* 2014

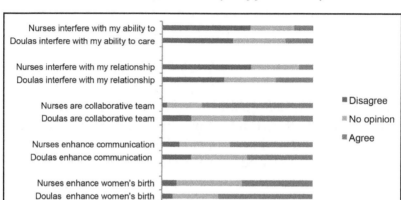

working with doulas, who as noted earlier, are present at a small percentage of all U.S. hospital births. About 20 percent of nurses disagreed that doulas enhance communication or are collaborative team members. Overall, both our survey and our qualitative data reveal nurses' cautiously supportive attitudes toward doulas: they like and appreciate doulas, but only if doulas stay within their labour-support role.

The imbalance between the nurses' role as hospital employee and the doula's role as invited guest as well as the overlapping boundaries of embodied care for birthing women may help explain why 73 percent of the doulas in the *Maternity Support Survey* agreed that "Nurses are collaborative team members" in contrast to the 46 percent of nurses who agreed that "doulas are collaborative team members." Doulas were also more positive about nurses than nurses were about doulas (55 percent of doulas compared to 43 percent of nurses agreed that the other role enhanced communication). Only 10 percent of doulas agreed that nurses interfere with the doula-client relationship, and 12 percent agreed that nurses interfere with doulas' ability to provide care to labouring women.

Because nurses' views of doulas were less positive than doulas' views of nurses, we looked for factors to help explain this disparity. We examined whether nurses thought insurance companies should cover doula services, and what aspect of the nursing role respondents enjoyed most: clinical care, labour support, or both equally. Unsurprisingly, we found that nurses who favoured insurance coverage were significantly more likely to have positive views of doulas than nurses who did not agree with insurance coverage for doula services. Nurses who said that they enjoyed clinical care the most (6.1 percent of the nurses) had the least favourable views towards doulas, whereas nurses who enjoyed labour support (21 percent of the nurses) had the most favourable views. Figure two displays the percentage of nurses who agreed or strongly agreed with the statements about doulas, by their preferred nursing role category.

Figure Two: Percentage of Nurses Who Agree with Statements about Doulas by Preferred Nursing Role, (N=893 Nurses), *Maternity Support Survey* 2014

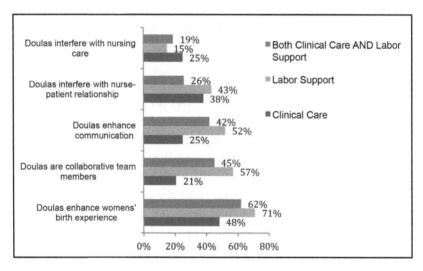

COLLABORATIVE LABOUR SUPPORT:
WHEN DOULAS MEET NURSES

Doulas cannot assume that nurses know what doulas are or have a complete understanding of doulas' scope of practice. Doulas enter institutionalized maternity care settings by virtue of their relationship with the birthing woman and know that their success in providing labour support is greatly facilitated when they cultivate collaborative relationships with labour and delivery nurses. Such success is contingent on the initial interactions of doulas and nurses, and on creating new relationships via ongoing negotiation with additional nurses who come on shift or replace the originally assigned nurse during her breaks.

Our qualitative data suggests that doulas report taking the initiative in establishing rapport with nurses as well as signaling their intention to work with the nurse, as a collaborative team, during labour:

> *My general rule is, I shake their hand, I say, "Hi my name is Kelly. I am so-and-so's birth doula. I am so happy to be here today and working with you as part of the birthing team." So I make it very clear that I am collaborative, and I'll talk with them, ask them questions, you know, find out if they have kids themselves, and I try to make that connection with them so they feel like I am a safe person to be around.* (Kelly, doula)

Kelly and other doulas understand that their role is to provide continuous labour support, whereas nurses provide clinical assessments and care for the mother-baby dyad. In interviews, doulas were very clear that they did not cross the line into providing medical care. Doreen, a doula, explained: "I am not doing anything medical as far as starting IVs or any of that kind of stuff. And I'm not messing with the monitors. I am there to give physical and emotional support only."

Nurses acknowledged that they are not usually able to devote significant amounts of their time to be with women throughout labour and recognized doulas' ability to provide continuous support. "I think [doulas] can come into the room and their agenda is to provide support to the woman through the whole process, whereas my agenda has to be, I have to chart on her hourly, you know, I have to make sure that the doctors are paged at this time and this time, so very different and very unique" (Heidi, Labor and Delivery (L&D) nurse). This ability to spend time with patients was echoed by the doulas as one of the ways their presence at a birth can benefit nurses and their clients. If someone knowledgeable and comfortable with labour is a continuous presence in the room, nurses do not have to check in as often and can focus on other aspects of their job. This was supported by Heidi, a L&D nurse, who said: "It's just nice to know that they have somebody who's in the room with them, like helping them with position changes, helping them get through early labour." And Tina, a L&D nurse noted, "A doula can really provide the labour support that we can't as a nurse because we have to do so much charting, unfortunately, but that's just the reality of health care."

OVERLAPPING BOUNDARIES: WHOSE CARE, WHOSE BODY?

The potential for overlapping boundaries between nursing and doula care arises when each member holds a certain position or lays claim to the same type of care for the birthing woman's body. Negotiation of roles and boundaries occurs each time nurses and doulas meet. One area of possible overlap concerns monitoring of the woman's birth plan. The nurses in our qualitative study reportedly had no problems with doulas who took a leading role in advocating for women's birth plans. Nurses said that they were comfortable with doulas helping the care providers remember what was on the woman's birth plan. As one nurse shared,

> *Sometimes we forget to remind patients that, no, they're not getting out of bed once they get the epidural. Sometimes the doulas are there to say, "But remember you wanted to be able to get out of bed and you're not going to be able to get out of bed if you get the epidural." (Jessica, L&D nurse)*

Since doulas are present throughout labour, nurses can rely on them as a continuous source of information about women's preferences.

Doulas express a willingness to take on particular tasks to overtly demonstrate to nurses that they were on the "same team." For example, doulas described how they work to appear as helpful as possible. Tamara, a doula, described how she tries to convey her role as one of helper:

*And I really try to help the hospital staff help the woman.
So if I could, you know, help her to get up to go to the
bathroom and we don't have to call the nurse, I share that
with the nurse. "Hey, put me to work. However you see
that I can help you, you know." And so I really try to just
create a synergy between all of us.* (Tamara, doula)

Tamara expresses a desire to help but also clarifies when her help
can be viewed as complementary to, rather than conflicting with,
the nursing role. If doulas clearly and successfully negotiate their
roles and activities with nurses, then when doulas assist a woman out of bed to the bathroom, it can be perceived by nurses as
helping. However, if the woman is on certain medications or in
the midst of a necessary fetal monitoring session, nurses may view
such actions by doulas as encroaching on their role, or a potential
patient safety issue.

OVERSTEPPING BOUNDARIES AND MISUNDERSTANDINGS

When doulas and nurses do not successfully negotiate boundaries
in terms of their respective labour-support roles, then overstepping
one's acceptable role and/or misunderstanding on both sides can
occur. In our qualitative data, most doulas did not see themselves
as typically overstepping boundaries but were very aware that
nurses often view doulas this way. Such overstepping was usually
described in terms of doulas' views on medical procedures and
medications.

Meredith, a doula, observed, "I definitely think they see doulas
as people who are anti-the medical establishment." Indeed, nurses
expressed frustration with doulas whom they had seen express
strong views about their client's desire to avoid surgical or medical procedures, as Jessica, a nurse, reported: "'No matter what,
refuse a C-section,' you know, I can't tell you how many times
I've heard that stupid statement. 'No matter what, refuse pain
meds.' No, no." Nurses, with their broader range of experience,
resist such blanket statements in regard to clinical treatment
options. Data from the *Maternity Support Survey* found that
doulas were more likely than childbirth educators or nurses to

express strongly held views on the need for, or appropriateness of, typical labour procedures such as epidurals or induction of labour (Roth et. al. 20).

For their part, doulas acknowledged that some doulas are confrontational but disagreed that this characteristic or behaviour is representative of all doulas. Michelle, a doula, reacted strongly to the implication that other, more extreme, doulas' views are similar to her own, sharing, "And I really resent when it's implied that I am just there to make sure she doesn't get an epidural despite the health of the baby and mother. Like, of course not. I think that is the most irritating thing I ever hear" (Michelle, doula). Other researchers have found that the spectre of the "bad" doula is ever present, and that doulas find themselves having to defend their own practice against this extreme "other" (Morton and Clift 190).

Nurses were uncomfortable with doulas whom they believed made attempts to take over the care of the woman by influencing medical decisions, overriding or refusing the suggestions of the hospital staff, or giving information that was contradictory to the information that they had given the patients. Consider Heidi's (a nurse) account of when and why conflict arises between nurses and doulas. "I think a lot of [conflict] is because they—the doulas—don't seem to work with us and they kind of want to take over the care of the patient versus work as a team. And a lot of that is not the medical model we're used to. We don't routinely use herbs in labour" (Heidi, L&D nurse). Heidi's comment that some doulas want to "take over the care of the patient" indicates her sense that this constitutes an "off-side" offense, not within the approved boundaries of the doula's labour-support role. In her view, nurses are the arbiter of what is in the medical model and what is not, and contrary to what doulas may say, approved medical treatment does not include "herbs."

Some nurses expressed discomfort when they perceived doulas to encroach on nursing or clinical roles. For new nurses who may not have seen many women desire un-medicated labours or who may not have experience in supporting such women, an encounter with an experienced doula can become conflictual or uncomfortable, as Tina recalled about an early encounter with a doula:

I felt kind of actually intimidated and I felt like she was trying to run the show. The doula would be giving the patient information, and it didn't feel that it was always the right information. I felt conflict usually with her. I don't know if it was just her, or if it was just me, starting there and not feeling very confident in my position.... I felt like a lot of conflict or things that I would say, she would say different things, or, you know, vice versa. (Tina, L&D nurse)

Thus, power differentials in the nurse-doula interaction can operate in either direction depending on the experience of the person in the doula or nursing role. Experienced doulas may inadvertently intimidate new nurses because of their greater knowledge of labour-support techniques. Experienced nurses may have little patience for new doulas who have a lot of questions and devalue the knowledge that they share with their clients.

DISCUSSION

Individually, people providing labour support all have constraints to some degree. Nurses and midwives have other responsibilities and often do not have enough time. Partners or spouses are often unprepared and too emotionally attached to the woman and the outcome to think clearly throughout the long and often stressful experience of labour. Doulas as institutional outsiders can be viewed as a threat to the institution, whereas doulas who are part of in-hospital programs may be seen as complicit with institutional practices and less able to serve as independent advocates for labouring women. Doula and nursing care can complement each other and provide the fullest support possible (Rosen 29). When doulas and nurses can distinguish their roles and work collaboratively, they can enhance a woman's birth experience (Deitrick and Draves 401).

For doulas and nurses to accomplish these goals in practice, some researchers have argued that doulas should be considered co-members of the health care team and that effective teamwork recognizes and accepts the different roles and responsibilities (Adams and Bianchi 13; Ballen and Fulcher 309). To improve collaborative care, nurses suggested to have doulas shadow a nurse as part of their doula training. Heidi, a nurse, thought this might help clarify the role of the doula. "So maybe that's one thing that I feel like [doulas organizations] could do better, is really making sure that doulas understand what the nurse's role is and maybe even having them shadow a nurse. When the doula understands what our role is, it works out a lot nicer for everybody" (Heidi, L&D nurse). Although Heidi suggested shadowing as a strategy to help doulas understand the nursing role, it could also have the effect of familiarizing nurses with doulas. As the interviews make clear, many nurses are not familiar with doulas or have had a bad experience that affected their attitude toward doulas in general.

One doula suggested educating nurses about the role of doulas in providing labour support. She noted that she gives a lecture on doulas and labour support at her local community college's nursing program on a regular basis. She explained, "Every semester, the nursing instructor has me come and speak to the students on what a doula does, what it would look like working with a doula in a hospital." These ideas for incorporating exposure to doulas and nurses during the educational process could go a long way in bridging the existing gaps in collaboration.

Educational efforts can only go so far, however, to ensure collaborative practice at any particular birth. One expert advises nurses to explain the sequence of events before admission and again before any procedures, and that information should be offered frequently and freely among the patient and her doula (Bowers 751). One way information sharing can facilitate collaboration is for doulas and nurses to assess each other's level of experience. When doulas and nurses are confronted with overlapping or conflicting roles and expectations, the variation in their work experience or discordant understandings of each other's roles can compound the challenges. Whereas research has found that older, more experienced nurses provided more labour support (Barrett and Stark 16), new nurses may not have been trained or have experience in supporting women with non-pharmacological techniques. Given the challenging lifestyle of being an on-call doula, and the other challenges in providing labour support, many more new doulas are currently practicing than experienced ones. Amy Gilliland, a doula trainer, has noted the phenomenon of "more new doulas than experienced ones," and requests that nurses "Be patient with the beginning doula and help her to learn how to treat you. She wants to do her best to get along with you while helping her client to have the best birth possible. She may ask more questions about procedures and provider preferences until she becomes familiar with your facility" (Gilliland "The Doulas Have Arrived"). Doulas can also use various strategies to assess nurses' interest in and willingness to support client goals for birth, since doulas cannot expect that the nurse assigned to her client will be collaborative and favourable toward labour support or know how to work with a doula. Charge nurses usually are well aware of individual staff nurses' attitudes about labour support, and they try, when possible, to assign supportive nurses to patients arriving with a doula and a birth plan specifying a desire for un-medicated birth.

Doulas who work in hospitals with a high rate of epidurals need to realize that the nurses who work in such hospitals may not know how to provide labour support because of lack of exposure to un-medicated birth. Doulas can view such situations as an opportunity to teach and model the labour-support behaviours that they want the nurses to engage in and understand. Some hospitals with high volumes of epidurals are using multi-disciplinary teams to train nurses in labour support techniques that can be helpful for patients with and without epidurals.

U.S. women report that their primary source of support in labour was their husband or partner or the nursing staff (Declercq, Sakala, Corry, Applebaum and Herlich 16) and give high ratings to all sources of support, including labour nurses, however, they are most likely to rate their doulas as "excellent" in terms of quality of care (Declercq, Sakala, Corry, and Applebaum 16). Even though some doula trainers caution that nurses may feel threatened by doulas encroaching on their labour support role, our findings suggest that nurses, at least those who enjoy labour support, have the most positive views of doulas.

Given recent U.S. efforts to reduce unacceptably high Caesarean section delivery rates (American College of Obstetricians and Gynecologists 693), and interest in the doula role to help accomplish this (Kozhimannil, Hardeman, Attanasio, Blauer-Peterson, and O'Brien e114; Kozhimannil, Attanasio, Jou, Joarnt, Johnson, and Gjerdingen e341), it is highly likely that doulas and nurses will meet more frequently in the future. Acceptable boundaries around labor support roles between nurses and doulas are not always self-evident and need to be negotiated with each clinical interaction. Nurses, depending on their views of their roles and the roles of doulas, may view doulas as potential sources of conflict during labour and birth. Although both nurses and doulas may agree on the value of embodied and emotional supportive care in labour, this may not be enough to create successful collaboration. Nurses and doulas need to be cognizant of the potential of overlapping boundaries in providing labour support as well as the varying levels of experience and interest each role brings to the birthing room so that both roles may work collaboratively and effectively together.

Acknowledgements: We thank the rest of the Maternity Support Survey research team for their contributions and thoughtful suggestions on this chapter, including Megan Henley, Louise Roth, and Miriam Naiman-Sessions.

WORKS CITED

Adams, Ellise and Ann Bianchi. "Can a Nurse and a Doula Exist in the Same Room?" *International Journal of Childbirth Education* 19.4 (2004): 12-15. Print.

American College of Obstetricians and Gynecologists. "Obstetric Care Consensus no. 1:Safe Prevention of the Primary Cesarean Delivery." *Obstetrics and Gynecology* 123.3 (2014): 693-711. Print.

Ballen, Lois, and Ann Fulcher. "Nurses and Doulas: Complementary Roles to Provide Optimal Maternity Care." *Journal of Obstetric, Gynecologic, and Neonatal Nursing* 35 (2006): 304-311. Print.

Barrett, Samantha and Mary Ann Stark. "Factors Associated with Labor Support Behaviors of Nurses. *The Journal of Perinatal Education* 19.1 (2010): 12-18. Print.

Bianchi, Ann and Ellise Adams. "Doulas, Labor Support, and

Nurses." *International Journal of Childbirth Education* 19.4 (2004): 24-30. Print.

Bogdan, Janet. "Care or Cure? Childbirth Practices in Nineteenth Century America." *Feminist Studies* 4 (1978): 92-99. Print.

Bowers, Beverly. "Mothers' Experiences of Labor Support: Exploration of Qualitative Research." *Journal of Obstetric, Gynecologic and Neonatal Nursing* 31.6 (2002): 742-752. Print.

Declercq, Eugene, Carol Sakala, Maureen Corry, and Sandra Applebaum. "Listening to Mothers II: Report of the Second National U.S. Survey of Women's Childbearing Experiences." *The Journal of Perinatal Education* 16.4 (2007): 15-17. Print.

Declercq, Eugene, Carol Sakala, Maureen Corry, Sandra Applebaum, and Ariel Herrlich. Deitrick, Lynn and Patrick Draves. "Attitudes Towards Doula Support During Pregnancy by Clients, Doulas and Labor-and-Delivery Nurses: A Case Study from Tampa, Florida." *Human Organization* 67.4 (2008): 397-406. Print.

Gilliland, Amy. "Beyond Holding Hands: The Modern Role of the Professional Doula." *Journal of Obstetric, Gynecologic and Neonatal Nursing* 31.6 (2002): 762-769. Print.

Gilliland, Amy. "After Praise and Encouragement: Emotional Support Strategies Used by Birth Doulas in the USA and Canada. *Midwifery* 27 (2011): 525-531. Print.

Gilliland, Amy. "The Doulas Have Arrived! Nurses, What Does this Mean for You?" *Doulaing the Doula*. n.p., 2014. Web. 20 Aug. 2014.

Hodnett, Ellen, Simon Gates, Justus Hofmeyr, and Carol Sakala. "Continuous Support for Women During Childbirth." *Cochrane Database of Systematic Reviews* 10 (2012): 1-113. Print.

Kozhimannil, Katy, Rachel Hardeman, Laura Attanasio, Cori Blauer-Peterson, and Michelle O'Brien M. "Doula Care, Birth Outcomes, and Costs Among Medicaid Beneficiaries. *American Journal of Public Health* 103.4 (2013): e113-121. Print.

Kozhimannil, Katy, Laura Attanasio, Judy Jou, Lauren Joarnt, Pamela Johnson, and Dwenda Gjerdingen. "Potential Benefits of Increased Access to Doula Support During Childbirth." *American Journal of Managed Care* 20.6 (2014): e340-e352. Print.

Leavitt, Judith. *Brought to Bed: Childbearing in America, 1750-1950*. Oxford: Oxford University Press, 1986. Print.

Morton, Christine, and Elayne Clift. *Birth Ambassadors: Doulas and the Re-emergence of Woman Supported Birth in America.* Amarillo, TX: Praeclarus Press, 2014. Print.

Rosen, Patricia. "Supporting Women in Labor: Analysis of Different Types of Caregivers." *Journal of Midwifery and Women's Health* 49.1 (2004): 24-31. Print.

Roth, Louise, Nicole Heidbreder, Megan Henley, Marla Marek, Miriam Naiman-Sessions, Jennifer Torres, and Christine Morton. *Maternity Support Survey: A Report on the Cross-National Survey of Doulas, Childbirth Educators and Labor and Delivery Nurses in the United States and Canada* (2014). *Research Gate.* Research Gate, 2014. Web. 1 Aug. 2014.

Torres, Jennifer. "Breast Milk and Labour Support: Lactation Consultants' and Doulas' Strategies for Navigating the Medical Context of Maternity Care." *Sociology of Health & Illness* 35.6 (2013): 924-938. Print.

Trevathan, Wenda. *Human Birth: An Evolutionary Perspective.* New York: Aldine de Gruyter, 1987. Print.

13.
Story-Centred Care

Full-Spectrum Doula Work and Narrative Medicine

ANNIE ROBINSON AND LAUREN MITCHELL

A S TWO FULL-SPECTRUM DOULAS and leaders of the Doula Project who met through our training in narrative medicine, our work is a daily symbiotic practice of both fields. We come to this work tied to the commitment of these archetypes of compassionate and narrative care: one of us has a background in radical mental health care, is an eating disorder recovery coach, and leads wellness programs for medical professionals and lay-people (AR); the other is a budding scholar of literature, medicine, and visual culture, and a former clinician in a high-risk hospital abortion clinic (LM). This essay reflects on the intersections of full-spectrum doula work and narrative medicine.

Just after 10:00 a.m. on a Friday, clad in ill-fitting scrubs, I (AR) situate myself beside Norita,[1] a petite 19-year-old Latina propped on a procedure table at the public city hospital. She is there to have an abortion; I am there as her doula, to support her through the experience. I know little about her, speak minimal Spanish, yet we organically join together as two bodies, two beings confronting and navigating this sensitive section of her story. Our eyes meet, and hers seize me: dark brown, they well with glassy tears, but remain resolute and strong. The doctor, a critical yet distant character in the scene, sweeps in and immediately becomes distracted and angry that the room where Norita will have her procedure is unprepared and not yet safe. I lock hands and eyes with Norita, establishing my steady presence. I begin breathing deeply, exhaling stresses of my own that do not belong in this room, and nod in encouragement as Norita begins to follow my lead. Instruments

clank at the bottom of the table as the doctor begins the procedure.
I clasp Norita's hand tighter and deepen our locked gaze, extend-
ing companionship, compassion, and affirming my commitment
to being with her as a collaborator in this narrative, embodied
experience of loss.

As full-spectrum doulas, we serve in a wide range of reproductive
health care settings in an effort to expand the birth doula model
of care to work with clients regardless of the outcomes of their
pregnancies. We see this work as inherently informed by and involved in co-constructing stories of the body. We endeavour here
to explicate the particularities of full-spectrum doula work, outline
what exactly narrative medicine is, and can do, and illustrate how
these two radical and transformative practices come together.

FULL-SPECTRUM DOULA CARE:
EMERGENCE, MISSION, AND PRACTICE

For the past forty years, doulas have been associated with the
"natural birth" movement, which picked up steam in the 1970s.
Birth doulas became gradually more prevalent in the 1980s as
Caesarean section rates increased and women felt the need for additional support to navigate the overuse of medical intervention in
obstetrical care.[2] In the twenty-first century, doulas have assumed
a place in common cultural knowledge. Their recent widespread
emergence has coincided with the development of the "birthing
justice" movement, a part of the reproductive justice movement,
which surpassed the natural birth movement in its focus on a
pregnant woman's right to birth alternatives, regardless of class,
gender identity, ethnicity, cultural orientation, religion, age, and
language.[3] Still, at this moment in time, when the word "doula" appears everywhere, from the literature of professional organizations
and conferences to pop culture references, it is usually associated
with birth. But there is a burgeoning segment of the doula world
that is challenging this limited association and incorporating doula
practice across the spectrum of pregnancy. This is known as the
full-spectrum doula movement.

The Doula Project, the first full-spectrum doula organization
in the country, was founded in 2007 in New York City. Its active

membership currently consists of a volunteer base of approximately 55 people who have collectively supported over 40,000 clients since 2008.[4] Although the founders of the formerly-named "Abortion Doula Project" began the organization expecting to emphasize abortions, they soon realized that the stories of their clients were deeply complicated. One often-told example is when one founder (LM) began to explain to a client, "When you have your *abortion* tomorrow..." but realized in seeing the look on the client's face and reading her contracted body language that something was wrong. She apologized, and the client began to tell her, "No, it's okay. You're right. That's what it is.... But we planned for this baby for so long, and he is sick. He doesn't have kidneys."

As an experience common to many doulas, this was the first of a series of moments in which the ability to listen, respond, and adjust care accordingly were bluntly underscored. The lesson was: "Mirror the language of your clients; do not name their procedure for them," which was a problem even in the original name of the organization. After we were asked to provide birth doula support for birth mothers who had made adoption plans, we changed our name to "the Doula Project," officially called ourselves full-spectrum doulas, and began to provide support at no cost to individuals across the spectrum of pregnancy choices, including during abortions, miscarriages, stillbirth inductions, adoption planning, and births for low-income individuals. We consider it imperative to offer support for all outcomes of pregnancy, especially because of how many people experience these outcomes and the stigma and silencing attached to them.[5]

The work of full-spectrum doula care differs in scope from traditional birth doula care insofar as we are not typically working with private clients: we partner with institutions themselves. In this public health model of doula care, we are explicitly dependent on the system for our ability to do this work. We graciously accept being granted access into these sterile, institutional facilities to partake in the most intimate of experiences as quiet, respectful caregivers. Offering support during these experiences in these settings can include chatting in the waiting room about the weather or their favourite television shows; practising deep breathing; reviewing their reasons for choosing this procedure; getting to know about their families, histories, work, and future dreams; offering hand massages and acupressure; or even just sitting with them in silence.

Full-spectrum doulas through the Doula Project must complete one twenty-four hour classroom training session where, as in most doula trainings, they are given a "bag of tricks." They are taught how to read body language, how to touch someone to provide physical comfort, how to provide emotional support by answering the hard questions that clients often ask, how to make small talk, and how to understand the procedure so that they may help their clients anticipate what to expect. Nonetheless, each doula has her own approach, and we see time and time again that the most important "quality" for a doula to have is an ability to act with sincerity, humility, and intuition. We see doulas who are able to provide support by saying and doing very little, by simply holding space for their clients, and others who are gregarious and turn to humour to make clients laugh a little if they can, even in a time of duress. But above all, the doulas must be malleable: we may each have our own style, but we are trained to listen to and adapt to our clients' needs.

A variety of motivations, interests, and expertise lead doulas to pursue training in full-spectrum care, including a proclivity for caregiving, a passion for social justice, a foundation in women's and gender studies, and an involvement in health care activism. Regardless of what drives their pursuit of this practice, all full-spectrum doulas must ask themselves—as we were once asked in a birth doula training—"Do you consider yourself a *birth* advocate? A *baby* advocate? Or a *woman* advocate?" The nuances seem slight but are in fact significant and essential for those of us devoted to providing non-judgmental, outcome-irrelevant support. We must stand firmly in the position as advocate for the client, the pregnant individual, first and foremost.

The Doula Project generally tries to avoid the use of gendered pronouns, and thus we use non-gendered language to state that we come to this work from the absolute perspective of *client*-centred advocacy—this is the very basis of the full-spectrum movement's mission. Other guiding tenets of the practice include the belief that our clients should be the leaders in their own care, and that all people are deserving and worthy of compassion, especially during times of vulnerability, conflict, or concern or, as we also often see, during experiences of joy, gratitude, and relief. We see the role of the doula as a well-trained caregiver, neither above nor below the client. We consider the doula an equal who stands in alliance with the client, working *within*, but *independent of*, the medical system. In effect, the doula is a guide and companion navigating through an often murky and unavoidably clinical journey. One of the greatest and most challenging lessons that we have learned is that we will never be able to take anyone's pain away, whether it be physical or emotional. But we can offer calm, professional clarity and grounding in times of great confusion and distress. Although the Doula Project initiated the conversation about "full-spectrum doula care," there are now many organizations that have taken the torch of this work. The role of organizations in full-spectrum doula care is to formalize the role of compassionate caregiver during any reproductive experience, to make it a regular part of clinic care, and thereby to create a "culture shift" within the spaces of reproductive health care.

NARRATIVE MEDICINE: NEED, EMERGENCE, AND APPLICATION

The art of telling stories and the art of deeply listening to stories were once central to the relationship between patients and clinicians. But in our contemporary health care system, those arts are often undervalued, as we tend to "privilege the biology over the biography" (Charon 121). This disconnect between patients and their caregivers can be repaired by promoting the role of telling and receiving stories within clinical interactions. Patients are more than bodies in need of treatment. They have stories that need to be heard. Practising narrative medicine in a clinic or hospital can facilitate better health care by ascribing value to the subjective experience of the patient, an aspect that is often lost in the objective stance, which dominates health care providers' training. Narrative medicine has been deemed "one of medicine's most important internal renovations" (Lewis 15) and is integral to humanistic approaches like doula care. We consider the principles and practice of narrative medicine to be the foundation on and materials out of which full-spectrum doula support is built.

Conceptually, defining the task of narrative medicine is not unlike the exercise that absorbed the six blind men and the elephant[6]: the practice of narrative medicine looks different to everyone who uses this model of care. Dr. Rita Charon, founder of the Program in Narrative Medicine, describes her practice as based in the act of listening to her patients with focus and without interruption. When she listens to her patients, her hands are still; she does not write notes, and she chooses her words carefully and sparingly to allow space for her patients to share their story. It is a patient, gentle practice. She also describes the act of "co-charting," which is a compassionate, supportive, and non-objective retelling of the entire story that she hears from her patient.

Dr. Sayantani DasGupta, another leader in the narrative medicine movement, correlates the clinician's practice, like the doula's practice, with what writers and readers do: all are "entering into (an experience) which necessarily resides outside (one's) own physical and emotional being (and) depends upon ... finding an entry point into that suffering from within her own imaginative self" (980). In other words, a clinician, or doula, enters into an unfolding story as a novelist does while writing a book and as a reader does while reading a book. As psychiatrist and writer Samuel Shem articulates, "the healing essence of narrative is not in the 'I' or the 'you,' but in the 'we'" (936). The powerful effects of attending to stories in health care depend on recognition of their collaborative construction.

Doulas, like the clinicians, must remember that although "we become invested in, wrapped up with, and, yes, coauthors of our patient's illness narratives ... we cannot ever claim to comprehend the totality of another's story" (DasGupta 980). DasGupta purports that the stance caregivers assume to "witness stories of suffering must be one of narrative humility" (980). We are to be compassionate guides, or companions, through an embodied experience. Our work as doulas has underscored the extent to which our cultural interpretation of empathy as a totalizing enterprise of completely understanding the experience of another person is unethical; to assume that it is possible to fully know the experience of another is projection, not empathy. We instead define empathy as the humility to recognize all that we do not know and to create space and patience to learn from our clients.

MERGING NARRATIVE PRACTICE AND DOULA CARE

The many complicated realities of doula care have proved to us the invaluable application of narrative medicine. This often occurs in the simple act of listening to how our clients choose to define themselves or their experiences. Doulas endeavour to offer explicitly non-judgmental support. But, of course, we are human and are prone to periods of strong feelings about the experiences of our clients. Our work is fraught with moments that are jarring: what do you do when a very sick patient with three children, for whom any pregnancy poses considerable risk to her health, is terminating her pregnancy because of sex selection and wants to try to become pregnant again? How do you attend to the needs of a patient who is enduring a pregnancy loss, but who is vocally angry at the other patients in the waiting room for having abortions? Or when your thirteen-year-old client doesn't want to use condoms or birth control because she doesn't think she will ever have sex again?

The practice of non-judgmental support means that, despite our personal thoughts and feelings—which we must continuously reflect on with as clear a mind and as open a heart as possible—we field our clients' questions and assuage their concerns, which are often fraught with anecdotes. Patients' personal anecdotes are perhaps the most powerful obstacle that the field of medicine must confront. No matter how specific the facts may be, it is the story that is personal. For example, if an IUD is supposed to be over 99 percent effective, but a client's sister got pregnant after getting one three years ago, it is difficult to try to convince her that an IUD is still, statistically, a reliable method of birth control. For medical providers working in defense of scientific fact and reasoning, who represent the hospital and all of its associated bureaucracy, moments when a patient counters medical fact with a singular anecdote are among the most frustrating.

As doulas, we are non-medical and are, therefore, largely exempt from the major responsibilities that affect a patient's health. This allows us access to a different interiority of patient narrative afforded by the flexibility of our professional parameters. Although we label ourselves "non-medical support people," we must acknowledge the extent a doula—just like any other non-medical health provider—can affect a patient's care. Doulas are not supposed to offer medical advice rather information. But because of the often highly interpretive nature of the medical field, it is hard for anyone to find wholly unbiased information. This is a key facet of narrative practice: the ways in which people seek out the information that supports the argument that they want to make. Doulas are quite privy to the ways in which narratives affect medical decisions, regardless of their medical veracity.

Because doulas are distanced from the mechanics of the procedure itself, and have no job other than to serve the client and the space, we are in an ideal position to provide narrative-based care. We can facilitate a narrative-based experience that transcends the traditional bio-medical experience by drawing attention to the subjective, storied experience that subsumes the physiological, objective one. For example, the medical provider asks the obligatory, "Do you have any questions about the procedure?" when the patient is already propped on the procedure table, clad in a paper gown, legs splayed in stirrups. In response, the patient clamps her lips shut and shakes her head no, although a swirl of emotions and thoughts are evident in her teary eyes and white-knuckled, clenched hands. Her questions and concerns may not pertain to the medical procedure itself, which has been explained to her during previous appointments. But the invitation to speak, to be known, is pertinent to her ability to be present for this experience and will ease later distress. To prevent the door of participation from being closed, the doula can offer her hand and gently ask, "What are you feeling right now?" or say, "This is a significant moment right now. I bet there are a lot of thoughts and feelings you're experiencing. That's totally normal. Do you want to share any of them with us?" We help the individual connect with the broader, non-medical narratives surrounding the procedure to include a more humanistic way of experiencing the situation at hand.

Attending to the narrative aspects of an abortion experience encourages an appreciation for the holistic experience of the abortion and can ease any traumatic, dehumanizing effects of the medical procedure for everyone involved.[7] Such gentle, humanistic questions can also be asked of the providers—before the queue of back-to-back procedures begins, during breaks between clients, or at the close of a long day. Fostering relationship and reflection through inquiry creates a meaningful pause amid the stress and flurry of the hard realities of the medical procedures that have the potential to disconnect and shut down both providers and patients. We feel compelled to provide whatever narrative care that we can to our providers almost as often as we do with our patients.

THE REALITIES OF CAREGIVING:
PLAYERS, CHALLENGES, AND APPROACHES TO CHANGE

Obstetrics and gynecology is an exhaustive and therefore exhausting field, which often "eats its own" in terms of provider care. Providers often work brutal hours to serve a large patient population with a huge diversity of needs. To that end, doctors are rarely able to attend to their own core needs, even as they are encouraging patients to eat well, sleep well, and to reduce stress in their lives. As doulas, we bear witness to the extensive burnout among the providers with whom we share space. They thus become additional subjects to whom we offer compassionate care. Their own stories of hardship, fatigue, and worry must, like their clients', be heard to optimize the process and outcomes of the medical procedures. In short, when the well-being of the providers is not tended to, everyone involved suffers.

Many providers internalize the triumphs and devastations of their clients: this is a result of the co-constructed narrative of provider and provided-for that unfolds in such intimate care. We have often witnessed providers walk into a day of procedures still feeling wounded by the questions or doubts in clinical judgment from the previous patient. Caregivers take their patients' decisions, and their pain, very personally. And thus, to protect themselves and their capacity to work, providers often begin to seek objectivity so much that the pain dissolves.

At the hospital where the Doula Project began its practice, author LM facilitated a workshop series as part of a study to determine the use of close reading and reflective writing sessions to assuage burn-out in OB/GYN residents.[8] While many of the residents do not identify as writers, when put to the task, most were able to beautifully articulate the tensions between coughing up statistics for patients and speaking to their individual needs. They discussed how terrifying it became to make mistakes, how little they felt that they knew, how tired they were, and how they often depended on partners and family for their emotional survival. They talked about the cases that kept them up at night: "Would the baby have survived if I had just done a C-section earlier? How can I make that doubt go away, when I go home and hold my own healthy children? Do I deserve to stop feeling guilty?"

In high-risk abortion care, doctors run across unique ethical and surgical dilemmas that have no roadmap. Most of the time, abortion is a very safe and straightforward procedure, but the times when it is not cause providers to feel very isolated. Residents are especially vulnerable to the pressures and concerns of caring for others, and they get some guidance from their attending physicians but with usually no larger conversation about the emotional burden of high-risk abortion.[9]

Late in the evening, I (LM) returned to the hospital after my shift to check on Valerie, one of my clients that day with whom I was especially close. The recovery room where I expected her to be was empty, and I was told she was still in surgery. My heart sank; that could only mean that there had been an emergency or complication.

Yesterday, Tara, the resident responsible for her care, and I looked into Valerie's panic-stricken face with assurance. "Nothing is ever 100 percent," we said, "but the likelihood of anything bad happening to you is low." We squeezed her hand and told her she would be fine, quoted statistics. We looked at each other with confidence. But today, dressed in the requisite uniform of scrubs, paper booties, and "bouffant cap," I walked into the strange, privileged space of the operating room with a tentative familiarity built only after years. I pushed a paper mask to my face and walked in, the space buzzing with nurses, doctors, techs, medical

*students. The attending physician and Tara looked up from over
the body of Valerie. Emergency hysterectomy.*

*"Phew," the attending sighed, "thank God you're here." She
sent Tara to scrub out of the case and switch with another resident. "Will you be able to stay with us for a while, until we're
done?" I nodded, surprised to have been regarded at all, feeling
useless during such devastating chaos. Tara and I walked out of
the room, and it was then I saw her eyes glassy with tears. I put
my hand on her shoulder, "I'm so sorry." There is so little that can
be said at these moments. We stopped in the hallway, my hand on
her shoulder while she wept. She was thirteen hours into her day,
had barely eaten, or gone to the bathroom. She was a raw nerve;
who wouldn't be?*

*It was likely that Valerie's hysterectomy was unavoidable, but
the hours before we would know for sure whether it was a uterine
abnormality or a provider mistake were long ones. Tara and I
hugged. Valerie's life had changed and she didn't know it yet. Tara
wanted to provide abortions to help people, not to cause so much
pain. We remembered our conversation from the day before. We
knew that we would be called on to reassure patients in the future
that their procedure is safe, that they shouldn't worry. But we knew
that with memories like this the task had become gargantuan.*

It is not uncommon for doulas to be sharp critics of the medi-
cal-industrial complex. Doulas regularly bear witness to challenging
moments, where we feel vulnerable or limited in our ability to
advocate against what may seem like problematic medical advice
from the perspective of non-medical providers. At the same time,
experienced doulas have accrued extensive knowledge about the
birth process, and many have seen the poor outcomes that occur
with poor patient support and the over-medicalization of obstetrical
care. We have met and been inspired by many providers at various
stages of their careers—nurses, attending physicians, counsellors,
residents, and medical students—the latter are especially prone to
emotionally attaching themselves to patients. Out of appreciation
and respect for these individuals, we take issue with a system that
fails to leave room enough for providers to care for their patients
in the way that they would ideally want to. A doula may serve as
a source of support for a resident navigating the overwhelming

burden of pursuing OB/GYN, which involves grappling with the strange emotional terrain of the surgery that is abortion or for a medical student realizing that despite their extensive education, this kind of care demands a very particular kind of support that converges at the fraught juncture of emotional, physical, and political confusion.

We grapple with nuanced perspectives based on our experiences in direct care. As we extend empathy to all constituents of these medicalized spaces and acknowledge that our clinical colleagues are doing the best that they can with scant resources, we find critique painful but necessary to give. We are not often able to consider what would be ideal; we work within a system that is filled with gritty reality and therefore have learned to balance our critique with empathy for the many people who provide exhausting levels of direct care work all day, every day.

LIVING IN THE SHADOW OF STORIES: SELF-CARE AND NARRATIVE HUMILITY

One critical implementation of narrative practice for doulas, ideally for all medical providers, is as a strategy for self-care. Doctor and educator Katharine Treadway has studied the effects of reflective practices on clinicians and believes "reflection that is integrated with clinical experience, not separate from it, is critical to ... professional and emotional growth" (Treadway and Chatterjee 1192). Writing and speaking one's story is a crucial way of handling and healing from vicarious trauma and compassion fatigue that caregivers experience, and it can be done in a multitude of ways. Individually, we employ narrative medicine by notetaking, journaling, even writing poetry and prose after shifts while always maintaining the confidentiality of our clients identifying information. We "story" by recounting our experiences in the clinic rooms one on one with fellow doulas and in groups of other doulas. By capturing in words, textual and oral, the often confusing, sad, and stressful experiences that we have, we are released from carrying them. Furthermore, our doubts about if we said or did the "right thing" can be assuaged and our worries and frustrations validated when others acknowledge that they have also encountered such circumstances. So too is it important that we share the joyful and even comical experiences we have, to refresh and remind us that there is no mono-story of loss. Our palettes thus cleansed after narrating, we may carry on with our lives outside of our doula work and return to the clinic at our next shift clear and grounded for the next round of life stories in which we will play a brief but meaningful role.

As previously mentioned, a crucial topic that we often confront in our caregiving as doulas—and consider in our critiques of healthcare delivery—is the practice of narrative humility. When we direct it toward *self-care*, it entails a commitment "to a lifelong process of self-evaluation and self-critique" (DasGupta 981). We must consider "our own role in the story, our expectations of the story, our responsibilities to the story, and our identifications with the story" (DasGupta 981).

Jasmin scarcely looked up from her phone when I (AR) introduced myself and led her into the procedure room to change into a scratchy paper gown. She was seventeen years old, heavily tattooed and pierced, and gnawed on her lower lip in evident agitation. She offered me a dismissive grunt when I asked if she had any questions. I sighed, silently, as I pulled the curtain closed to give her some privacy while changing. I worried I might not be able to connect with her as closely as I wished I could.

Once changed, Jasmin twitched her right foot as she sat on the edge of the hard table. I took a seat on the low wheeled stool before her and looked into her stormy grey eyes that briefly glanced into my own. I asked her how she was feeling, who was waiting for her outside, how her day had been. She only gave slight shrugs and murmurs in response. "What can I do right now?" I searched my mind and scanned my instincts for an answer. "How can I best support her in this moment? What might she want from me?" But before I could attempt any other tactics, the medical team burst into the room.

As the nurse administered her sedative medication through the IV in her left arm, I took Jasmin's right hand in mine. She surprised me by squeezing it in appreciation, and I humbly realized the need to suspend the assumptions I had made—that she didn't like me, that she felt my presence superfluous and unhelpful, and that her distant demeanour conveyed a desire to be left alone. I could relate to her more than I had initially thought. I, too, sometimes acted irritability and pushed others away when frightened and vulnerable. I smiled to her and to myself, as I caressed her hand.

Moments later, once the medication had taken effect and the procedure was underway, she jolted her head towards me and began recounting to me in a jarringly loud voice traumatic events from her childhood. She asked me if I'd ever been sexually abused or hit, if I knew what she was going through. I held fast to her hand and tried my best to keep up with her lines of questioning, aware that this sudden animation was probably a strong reaction to the disinhibiting medication. Although she most likely would not remember exposing these most intimate stories to me once the effects wore off, I needed to be there for her in this moment in the most sensitive and nurturing way I could.

Although I could not personally relate to the horrors Jasmin told me about, I could try to guide her through the emotions she was exhibiting. I held fast to her hand and maintained our locked eyes, nodded when she sought validation. As I witnessed her pain— physiological discomfort from the procedure, psychological and emotional distress from the memories—I offered her unwavering presence and comfort: that was the best I could do as she unloaded unrelatable yet vivid and meaningful tales to me.

We must "recognize that each story we hear holds elements that are unfamiliar" and honour that these unfamiliar aspects may in fact be the "most valuable nuances and particularities" (DasGupta 981) in our client's experience, and by acknowledging and honouring them we are granting her an attention and validation that she may otherwise not receive in this clinical encounter. DasGupta asserts that her notion of narrative humility—and we would argue the practice of narrative in clinical encounters in general—"approaches what has been called mindfulness in medicine" (981). Such an approach allows us all—doulas, clinicians, and clients alike—to reconfigure our relationships to the medical procedure, to one another other, and to our own self. This reconfiguring, we believe, is an essential, radical, and transformative way of caregiving and being in the world as embodied, interconnected human beings.

DOULA CARE, NARRATIVE CARE: TO LOVE THE OTHER

Our work is defined by the stories of others, and as doulas it is our role to be patient and vigilant listeners, to be malleable in our practice, and to allow the clients to determine how they wish to receive care. Within the exhausted field of medicine, wherein patients internalize the effects of the problematic system, the doula's role is to work within the system but differentiated from it, which means that we are able to honour story above all. We bear witness to the experience of others; we assist in and support the creation of the client's story. And these stories, in turn, become co-constructed artifacts within the doula's provider narrative. Likewise, we are dependent on our own narratives within our practices of self-care to help clarify our experiences and make sense of them. In its ultimate essence of unflinching bearing witness to loss, love, joy, relief, and sorrow, doula care is synonymous with narrative practice and provides our clients, our provider colleagues, and one another with the reminder: "You are strong, you are brave, and you deserve to feel beloved."

ENDNOTES

[1]Names have been changed to protect clients' identities.
[2]See especially: Gilliland. Also see: Klaus and Kennell; Trainor.
[3]This sea change has been inspired by current, often unpublished or non-scholarly, work of activists on the ground. Conference culture has been a huge player in the development of activist communities who seek to push boundaries of care and justice. Most specifically, the Civil Liberties and Public Policy (CLPP) Annual Conference, "From Abortion Rights to Social Justice" began to regularly feature doulas and midwives as speakers. In 2006, NPO National Advocates for Pregnant Women held the first major conference of its kind meant to explicitly bring in activists and medical communities who were interested in the rights of pregnant people, whether they chose to continue the pregnancy or not. These conferences played key roles in the inspiration of the Doula Project.
[4]Most recent numbers derived from the Doula Project internal

records as of November 2014. Numbers published in annual fundraising appeal at the end of the fiscal year (December 2014). [5]We would like to thank and support the work of our fellow organizations who have been a huge inspiration to the Doula Project, particularly Backline and Exhale. Exhale has been spearheading the "Pro-Voice" movement, aimed to provide an apolitical safe space for people who have experienced abortion.

[6]An old fable in which each "blind man" touches a different part of an elephant's body and "sees" it to be something else, with no two interpretations being alike.

[7]Our experience has clarified for us the extent to which all surgery is often as much of a traumatic or dehumanizing event as it is a positive one. Our clients are not unilaterally traumatized by their procedures, and as we know, every experience looks and feels different. But, what we will say is that medical procedures are stressful, and it is extremely rare that we would come across a client who was not apprehensive at the thought of a surgery, no matter how safe it is.

[8]Manuscript entitled "Using Structured Reflection to Understand Factors Contributing to Burnout and Support Humanism in OBGYN Residents," by Winkel, et.al. Under review; publication forthcoming 2015.

[9]For further reference, see Grimes.

WORKS CITED

Charon, Rita. "Narrative Medicine as Witness for the Self-telling Body." *Journal of Applied Communication Research* 37.2 (2009): 118-131. Print.

DasGupta, Sayantani. "Narrative Humility." *The Lancet* 371.9617 (2008): 980-981. Print.

Gilliland, Amy L. "Beyond Holding Hands: The Modern Role of the Professional Doula." *Journal of Obstetric, Gynecologic, & Neonatal Nursing* 31.6 (2002): 762–769. Print.

Grimes, David. "The Continuing Need for Late Abortions." *JAMA* 280.8 (1998): 747-50. Web. 16 Nov. 2015.

Lewis, Bradley. "Narrative Medicine and Healthcare Reform." *Journal of Medical Humanities* 32.1 (2011): 9-20. Print.

Klaus, M. H. and J. H. Kennell. "The Doula: An Essential Ingredient of Childbirth Rediscovered." *Acta Pædiatrica* 86.10 (1997): 1034-1036. Web.16 Nov. 2015.

Shem, Samuel. "Fiction as Resistance." *Annals of Internal Medicine* 137:11 (2002): 934-937. Print.

Treadway, Katharine and Neal Chatterjee. "Into the Water - The Clinical Clerkships." *The New England Journal of Medicine* 364.13 (2011): 1190-1193. Print.

Trainor, Cynthia L. "Valuing Labor Support."*AWHONN Lifelines* 6.5 (2002): 387–389. Web. 16 Nov. 2015.

14.
Between Two Worlds

Doula Care, Liminality, and the
Power of Mandorla Spaces

COURTNEY EVERSON AND MELISSA CHEYNEY

I N RECENT YEARS, A GROWING CALL for the support of normal, physiologic birth practices has developed in the United States in response to the negative maternal-infant health outcomes and experiences of disempowerment described by women as birth has become increasingly medicalized (American College of Nurse Midwives [ACNM], Midwives Alliance of North America [MANA], and National Association of Certified Professional Midwives [NA-CPM]; Amnesty International; Declercq et al.; Hamilton et al.). In 2013, the U.S. Caesarean section rate was 32.7 percent, more than two to three times what is estimated to be safe for women and babies (Hamilton et al.; Althabe and Belizán). Furthermore, the United States ranks thirty-third on the 2015 Mother's Index—a global index that evaluates the overall well-being of mothers and children by nation (Save the Children). Tragically, the U.S. lags behind despite the fact that the United States spends more than any other nation per capita on maternity care (Amnesty International). Add to this women's narratives describing dehumanization, victimization, and disempowerment in childbirth, and a clear need for a more nuanced conversation around maternity care reform emerges (Machizawa and Hayashi; Wagner).

Both doula care and homebirth midwifery have arisen as movements focused on re-humanizing childbirth via the support of normal physiologic birth and women's autonomy in birth place decision making. As such, they serve as cultural windows into the contentious arena of maternity care reform and place of birth debate discourses. However, these movements—seemingly allied in many core beliefs—have not always operated in solidarity. This disconnect may be tied to their differential locations within the obstetric hierarchy. While homebirth midwifery remains highly contested in the place of birth debate (Cheyney, Everson, and Burcher; Sandall, McCandlish, and Bick) doulas, in contrast, are at once intimately part of, and marginalized within, the obstetric community (Emad; Morton and Clift; Norman and Rothman).

In this chapter, we explore doula care as a *mandorla* space between hospital-based obstetrics and homebirth midwifery to examine how the liminal position of doulas allows for the negotiation of power and resistance within U.S. childbirth reform. Here we define liminality as a ritualized, transitional space located between two states of being (Turner; van Gennep), and a mandorla space as "the almond-shaped segment that is made when two circles partly overlap" (Johnson 98). As Johnson and Davis-Floyd argue in their use of the mandorla to examine home to hospital transfers, "inside the overlap, separate domains are united and merged into innovative structures, within which effective solutions can emerge" (472). Drawing on this conceptualization of the mandorla, we argue that although doulas primarily work within the obstetric system, their tacit threat lies in the recognition that doula care can constitute a vital common ground—and perhaps a critical opening—in larger place of birth and maternity care reform debates.

BACKGROUND:
MIDWIFERY, DOULA, AND MEDICAL MODELS OF CARE

In 1982, sociologist Barbara Katz Rothman outlined the essential elements of what she deemed the "midwifery model" of care, contrasting this model with the "medical model" and arguing that the fundamental differences in these two approaches to birth matter deeply for a woman's transition to motherhood. At the heart of the differences are opposing views on the mother-fetus relationship. Throughout this paper, we pluralize the term "model" to acknowledge the diversity existing within varying childbearing models of care, including midwifery, medical, and doula. In midwifery models, the mother and fetus are viewed as an "organic whole" (Rothman 276) or a symbiotic dyad, whereas in medical models, the mother and fetus are viewed as separate entities engaged in a parasitic or competitive relationship. Midwifery models position mothers as autonomous decision makers, in contrast to more patriarchal, medical models where physicians, by virtue of their ascribed knowledge and power, hold ultimate decision-making authority.

In 1992, anthropologist Robbie Davis-Floyd expanded Rothman's earlier work and proposed the "wholistic" and "technocratic" models of birth. The wholistic approach is woman-centred with family as a significant social unit; with woman as active subject; mother and child as one; home as nurturing environment; and bodily, experiential, and emotional knowledge as highly valued. Childbearing is understood as a healthy, normal process best supported by low-tech, high-touch techniques with a midwife as "skillful guide" (Davis-Floyd 160-161). Technocratic models, in contrast, are male-centred with social support regarded as unimportant or secondary to primary clinical concerns; with woman as passive object; hospital as "factory" and babies as "products"; and technical, scientific knowledge as the only knowledge of value. Childbearing is understood as dysfunctional, even pathological, and best controlled by interventions led by an obstetrician as "manager/skilled technician" (Davis-Floyd 160-161).

Collectively, Rothman and Davis-Floyd's work with care models has provided a key platform for U.S. childbirth movements today, essentially allowing disparate sides of maternity debates to identify with and rally around one approach, while using the opposing model to distance the other. Moreover, these models have frequently been aligned with distinct places of birth—midwifery models with home and birth centres, and medical models with hospitals. Importantly, when Rothman first conceived of and named these juxtaposed models, she intentionally did not name them with respect to site of delivery, claiming that such a move would be "too restricting" (25). "Doctors can bring the medical model right into the home ... And a midwife can bring much of the alternative [midwifery] model into the hospital" (25). It is this potential for overlap that allows for the production of liminality in the performativity of doula care—a conceptual mandorla space, at once betwixt and between. Situated within the in-between, doulas may find themselves metaphorically and theoretically stateless, between two worlds, suspended in limbo. However, they may also capitalize on the ritual power of the in-between (Turner; Rayner) and, in so doing, expose conceptual spaces where dominant bio-medical discourses of childbirth may be challenged.

METHODS

In order to identify and describe the position of doulas within the U.S. maternity care landscape, we combined content analysis (Creswell; Hays and Singh) of published literature on doula pro-fessional standards, core competencies, scopes of practice, and care philosophies (table one) with extensive participant observation. We reviewed literature from three national childbirth/doula professional organizations—Childbirth and Postpartum Professional Associ-ation (CAPPA), Doulas of North America (DONA) International, International Childbirth Education Association (ICEA)—and two maternity care advocacy organizations—Lamaze International (Lamaze) and Childbirth Connection (CC)—who have published materials that met two criteria: 1) the publicly available document describes the scope and intended impact of doula care; and 2) the document is designed to reach a national audience (i.e., they are not documents created for a specific doula practice or hospital-based program). Each of the selected texts was systematically analyzed for emergent themes by using consensus coding of core values and concepts (i.e., *in vivo* codes) that reoccurred across multiple documents (Creswell; Hays and Singh). Our goal was to identify essential elements of doula care models as formalized in official documents and position statements, which could then be discussed and interpreted through the lens of our own lived experiences of researching, observing, and providing doula and midwifery care over the last fifteen years.

We also re-examined field notes collected during multisite ethno-graphic research with both homebirth midwives and doulas. Our dual positionalities as a birth doula and medical anthropologist (Everson), and a homebirth midwife and medical anthropologist (Cheyney), have allowed for extensive participant and contribut-ing observation (Creswell; DeWalt and DeWalt) across multiple models of care and birth settings (home, hospital, and birth centre)

Table One: Documents analyzed for content analysis of the essential elements of doula care models

Organizational Author		Document(s) Title
Professional Doula Organizations	Childbirth and Postpartum Professional Association (CAPPA)	•CAPPA Position Paper: Evidence-based Labor Doula Care •Labor Doula Scope of Practice Available at: www.cappa.net.
	Doulas of North America International (DONA)	•DONA Position Paper: The Birth Doula's Contribution to Modern Maternity Care •Birth Doula Standards of Practice Available at: www.dona.org.
	International Childbirth Education Association (ICEA)	•ICEA Position Paper: The Role and Scope of Birth Doula Practice •ICEA Position Paper: Physiologic Birth Available at: www.icea.org
Childbirth Advocacy Organizations	Childbirth Connection	•Childbirth Connection's Pregnancy Topic on Labor Support: Resources for Labor Support during Pregnancy and Childbirth / Available at: www.childbirthconnection.org
	Lamaze International	•Healthy Birth Practice #3: Bring a Loved One, Friend, or Doula for Continuous Support / Available at: www.lamazeinternational.org.

as well as at numerous professional conferences, birth worker meetings, community outreach events, and legislative hearings and rallies. Throughout these activities, we have spoken formally and informally with dozens of midwives, doulas, and physicians about their professional philosophies, care beliefs, and attitudes towards maternity care reform.

This combination of content analysis and participant observation enabled us to situate the results of our textual inquiry against the backdrop of larger childbearing belief systems, relying on Davis-Floyd's and Rothman's conceptualization of technocratic/ medical and holistic/midwifery models as guiding frameworks. Collectively, our findings help to characterize the intersections and discordances between medical and midwifery paradigms—a mandorla space where, we argue, mothers and doulas engage in forms of resistance that challenge dominant biomedical discourses of childbirth and reveal the potential for systems-wide transformation.

RESULTS: (RE)CONCEIVING DOULA MODELS OF CARE

In the pages that follow, we describe five themes that emerged from our analyses and that, we argue, form the core components of doula care models: 1) specialists in the psychosocial needs of childbearing women; 2) support of physiologic birth; 3) provision of individualized, evidence-based support; 4) facilitation of communication and relationship; and 5) continuous companionship. These key themes form the essential elements of doula models of care while also revealing both the liminal nature of the mandorla space created between childbearing paradigms (medical and midwifery) and the negotiation of doula models within it.

Theme One: Specialists in the Psychosocial Needs of Childbearing Women

Doulas—as non-medical labour support companions—have largely carved out their niche on the maternity care team through their emphasis on the psychosocial needs of childbearing women. Position papers and scopes of practice set forth by professional doula and advocacy organizations extensively discuss the significant emotional and social aspects of birth. As DONA explains, "Perhaps the most crucial role of the doula is providing continuous emotional reassurance and comfort for the entire labor" (1). The core of this emotional support dimension lies in the commonly repeated phrase "mothering the mother" (Childbirth Connection; Klaus), meaning that the doula aims to serve as a calm and nurturing presence who provides the woman with the emotional reassurance and encouragement to birth from a position of confidence. As CAPPA notes, "they [laboring women] require emotional support, information, reassurance, encouragement, respect and love ... a labor doula can meet many of these non-medical needs" ("Position Paper" 1). Birthing with support—and the experiences of nurturing care received—then translates into improved confidence in parenting and enhanced bonding between mother and baby. CAPPA states, "One of the most important roles of the labor doula is to attend to the mother's emotional needs during labor, birth, and immediate postpartum as positive emotional care can strengthen bonding with her infant" ("Position Paper" 1). DONA similarly echoes the importance of emotional support and its translation to enhanced parenting: "The quality of emotional care received by the mother during labor, birth and immediately afterwards is one vital factor that can strengthen or weaken the emotional ties between mother and child" (1).

Childbirth is constructed in these documents as a highly psychosocially and spiritually open period for women, and memories of the birth are believed to affect self-image and parenting behaviours of the new mother throughout her life. As CAPPA explains,

> Having a baby is an experience that is remembered forever by the woman and her family ... the way a birth unfolds will affect a woman's confidence as a person and mother, her self-esteem, and her relationships with others. ("Position Paper" 1)

These memories are influenced by the emotional support obtained. Lamaze asserts, "One of the most important roles a doula plays is to help you have the best possible memory of your birth" (2). Doula care, thus, is intended to support and enhance the positive psychosocial aspects of birth, while mitigating those that induce stress. In Childbirth Connection's words, "Labor is an intense physical and emotional experience. It's comforting to be reassured that what's happening is normal and healthy and to get feedback about your progress in labor." When psychosocial needs are met, labour is allowed to progress uninterrupted, which, in turn, facilitates normal, physiologic birth.

Theme Two: Support of Physiologic Birth

Doula models of care espouse an understanding of birth as a physiologic, rather than a purely medical, process; in CAPPA's words, "Childbirth is not simply a medical event" ("Position Paper" 1). Normal, physiologic childbearing is described as "one that is powered by the innate human capacity of the woman and fetus" (ACNM, MANA, and NACPM 2), meaning that birth is allowed to unfold without interventions that may disrupt underlying physiologic mechanisms and processes. As ICEA defines it: "Physiologic birth is a birth where the baby is birthed vaginally following a labor which has not been modified by medical intervention" ("Position Paper: Physiologic Birth" 1). Doula models of care aim to support physiologic birth through physical and emotional comfort measures during labour that promote cervical dilation and fetal decent, and that help to avoid the cascade of interventions that disrupts normal birth. ICEA explains that "a doula physically supports the mother in a variety of ways. She will suggest alternative (upright and gravity positive) positions for the mother, remind her to maintain her fluid intake, make sure she goes to the bathroom frequently, or offer the use of heat/cold therapy for stress and pain relief" ("Position Paper: The Role and Scope" 2). Similarly, CAPPA states, "She [the doula] will assist the mother and her partner to find the best methods to relax and encourage labor, including helping with maternal position change, breathing, relaxation, imagery, massage, acupressure, and other comfort measures" ("Position Paper" 1). DONA echoes, "The doula offers help and advice on comfort measures such as breathing, relaxation, movement and positioning, and comforts the woman with touch, hot or cold packs, beverages, warm baths and showers, and other comforting gestures" (1).

Lamaze International and Childbirth Connection both highlight research on the benefits of continuous labour support measures—citing the Cochrane Reviews (Hodnett et al.) as the best evidence to date—wherein women without continuous labour support were more likely to: use an epidural, other "regional" analgesia, or other medications (including narcotics) to manage pain; give birth via Caesarean section or assisted with vacuum extraction or forceps; give birth to a baby with a low five-minute Apgar score; and be dissatisfied with or negatively rate their childbirth experience (Childbirth Connection). The physical comfort measures doulas administer—in tandem with support of psychosocial needs—provide a foundation for facilitating normal physiologic birth, an evidence-based approach to achieving safe and healthy births for all women.

Theme Three: Provision of Individualized, Evidence-based Support

Individualized and evidence-based care strategies are the central tenants of the educational support dimension provided by doulas. ICEA notes that "the doula should offer evidence-based information in a manner as unbiased as possible. Referring the client to reliable sources so that she can make her own decisions imparts confidence that she can draw upon during labor ... [doulas] provide information that helps the woman make informed decisions in conjunction with her healthcare providers" ("Position Paper: The Role and Scope" 1-2). Similarly, DONA echoes the educational support role of doulas: "The doula helps her [the mother] to become informed about various options, including the risks, benefits and accompanying precautions or interventions for safety" (2). Resources and educational guidance assist a mother in learning about perinatal health and parenting practices and, in turn, facilitate feelings of empowerment and mothering confidence.

Furthermore, the provision of evidence-based educational support occurs within an individualized context where culturally safe practices are honoured, or as ICEA writes: "A doula provides culturally appropriate emotional support to the laboring woman, helping her to cope with labor in her own way. The doula, as a servant, lays aside any preconceived ideas she may have and supports the mother in the way that the mother chooses to labor" ("Position Paper: The Role and Scope" 2). In doula models of care, each mother and her family are recognized as unique, holding values and desires for their birth that distinctly fit their life contexts and worldviews. As CAPPA explains, "Each woman will have different needs, both medically and emotionally due to her individual situation and desires" ("Position Paper" 1). DONA echoes these sentiments: "They [pregnant/laboring women] need individualized care based on their circumstances and preferences" (1). In response, doulas work to provide such individualized care and assist a mother in integrating evidence-based information with her own personal beliefs and values. Central to this theme is the recognition that individualized support means support of the mother regardless of what the doula might choose for herself, and no matter how the birth ends up unfolding. As ICEA explains, "Since the core of the doula's belief is to make this the very best birth experience for a woman, the doula can be a benefit regardless of the particular circumstances surrounding a birth" ("Position Paper: The Role and Scope" 2).

Theme Four: Facilitation of Communication and Relationships

Respect for a woman and her family's individualized needs and desires can be communicated to other members of the birth team with the goal of facilitating multiple relationships during the childbearing experience. Doula models aim to enhance communication between the mother and her health care providers—that is, not speaking "for women," but supporting the mother as she self-advocates for her own unique birth preferences. As DONA explains, "The doula helps ensure that these nonmedical needs are met while enhancing communication and understanding between the woman or couple and the staff" (2).

Doula models, thus, seek to nurture collaborative birthing environments by helping to make childbearing wishes known to all members of the maternity care team, or as CAPPA notes: "She [the doula] facilitates and promotes self-advocacy, informed choice, and effective communication between the family and care providers. She [the doula] seeks to foster a cooperative, respectful and positive atmosphere with all members of the birth team so that the mother can birth with confidence" ("Scope of Practice"). The doula encourages the mother to ask questions about her care, express her wishes, and elicit further clarification as the pregnancy, labour, and birth progress. When unexpected occurrences arise, the doula works with the mother to negotiate changes in a way that respects the mother's overarching needs, or in Lamaze's words: "If your labor takes a different path than expected, a doula can help you sort out your feelings and discuss your choices" (2). ICEA echoes, "In many cases, when clients have questions about medical issues, the doula can consider it an opportunity to facilitate communication between the client and her caregivers" ("Position Paper: The Role and Scope" 2). Similarly, Childbirth Connection asserts, "She [the doula] can also help you communicate your needs to hospital staff and support decisions that you and your partner have made." This ability to successfully advocate for the mother's individualized wishes arises largely from the ongoing nature of the relationship—a relationship of intimate and continuous support that is difficult or impossible to achieve by other members of the care team.

Theme Five: Continuous Companionship

Continuity of care is an essential and distinctive element of doula models of care, and conceptual definitions of the "birth doula" are frequently modified by the word "continuous." DONA, for example, defines a doula's primary task this way: "Doulas provide continuous physical and emotional support and assistance in gathering information for women and their partners during labor and birth" (1), while ICEA succinctly states: "A doula provides continuous care" ("Position Paper: The Role and Scope" 2). Professional organizations and advocacy groups consistently speak to the importance of continuous support for safe and healthy physiologic birth. Indeed, "continuous support" is among the six *Healthy Birth Practices* documented by Lamaze (Lamaze International, Green, and Hotelling) and, as CAPPA explains, "Labor doulas improve the outcome, both medically and emotionally, for the mother and her partner as well as the baby. One of the most critical roles of the labor doula is providing continuous reassurance, comfort, and emotional support during labor and birth" ("Position Paper" 4). ICEA further echoes this stance: "Continuous labor support has been shown to have positive pregnancy outcome benefits ... ICEA, therefore, believes that birth doula care should be available to every woman who needs or wants continuous labor support" ("Position Paper: The Role and Scope" 3).

Although labour support can and should come from a variety of sources—including partners, family/friends, nurses, doctors, and midwives—doula models claim that doulas play a distinct role in their ability to provide knowledgeable and continuous support. Because of the benefits attributed specifically to the continuous care provided by doulas, Childbirth Connection contends that "a trained labor support specialist is likely to be your best option for optimal labor support." They go on to explain that although family and friends, for example, may be able to provide consistent support, they may not be able to provide maximum benefits for several reasons, including: inexperience with support measures; uncertainty about the physiology of labour/birth; impact of (fear-based) media discourses; and difficulties with providing care in an unfamiliar environment (Childbirth Connection). Similarly, CAPPA claims that doulas and family/friends/partners hold complementary, but unique, roles: "The partner... knows the mother intimately and possesses a love that can come from no one else. The labor doula can offer unique help to the partner and friends by providing suggestions for him/her, and allow the partner, loved ones, and friends to participate at their comfort level" ("Position Paper" 2).

Additionally, health care providers may all desire to provide continuous support to labouring women, but they often hold other obligations—not the least of which is ultimate attention to and responsibility for the clinical outcomes of birth. As DONA explains, "Medical providers must assess the condition of the mother and fetus, diagnose, and treat complications as they arise, and focus on the safe delivery of the baby. These priorities rightly take precedence over the nonmedical psychosocial needs of laboring women" (2). Childbirth Connection cites three primary reasons why hospital-based providers and staff face barriers in providing optimal support, including: lack of education in labour support techniques; responsibility to other clients, tasks, and clinical monitoring; and shift disruptions that inhibit continuous and personalized support. Because of such institutionalized constraints as well as barriers faced by friends/family, Lamaze asserts that "many women find hiring a doula is the best way to ensure they will have continuous labor support" (2).

DISCUSSION:
LIMINALITY AND MANDORLA SPACES IN DOULA CARE

Collectively, these five elements outline a doula model(s) of care that fulfill(s) a unique and complementary role on the maternity care team, one of continuous companionship that is specialized, individualized, and grounded in the intertwined physiologic and psychosocial needs of childbearing women. As Rothman notes, "Birthing is something that women can do, but usually require emotional support and teaching to do well—that is, to the mother's own satisfaction" (181). Arguably, the targeted social support dimensions provided by doula care can occur in any site of delivery—home, birth centre, or hospital—and with any primary clinical care provider in attendance—midwife or obstetrician. As such, doulas can provide support to all families regardless of provider type, delivery site, birth wishes, or perinatal occurrences, but, concurrently, the very nature of this fluidity leaves them betwixt and between, neither fully belonging to homebirth midwifery nor hospital-based obstetrics—enter the mandorla space (figure one).

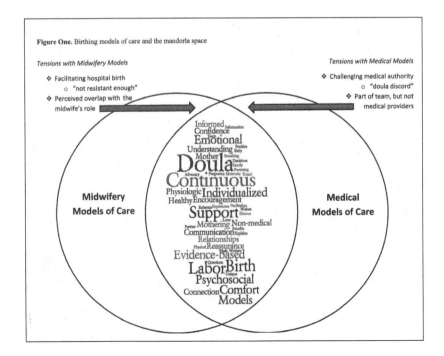

Figure One. Birthing models of care and the mandorla space

Within the mandorla space that doula models of care occupy, elements of each of the parent circles (midwifery and medical care models, respectively) are represented. Here, the continuity of space and fluidity of boundaries allow each source to flow into and out from the other as dynamically distinct, but not definitively discrete (Rayner). The mandorla is, thus, a liminal space—a threshold—where symbolism is received by the transitional being, or "liminal persona" (Turner 47), as they make the passage from one state of being to another. This liminality allows for transformation, dissolution, or reversal of social orders, traditions, and cultural paradigms (Turner). We argue, then, that doulas serve as a type of transitional birthing professional, mediating between the two parent models of care that engulf and press against the mandorla. Doulas hold open a space where the power of the in-between may be co-opted and used to instigate social transformation. But, how is this in-between generated and how can it be operationalized as a form of resistance?

Tension with Hospital-based Obstetrics

Doulas primarily find work supporting families that choose to birth in the hospital, often with obstetricians (Declercq et al.; Morton and Clift). In large part, this is due to current U.S. birthing culture where only about one percent of all births occur outside the hospital (MacDorman, Matthews, and Declercq). As such, doulas are at once intimately part of, and marginalized within, the obstetric hierarchy. Although doulas operate primarily within hospital-based obstetrics underscored by a medical/technocratic model, they find many intersections with the midwifery/holistic model of care, grounding their beliefs in the emotional and physiologic needs of childbearing women. Yet doulas do not—and likely cannot—outright reject technocratic birth because they rely on good relations with medical staff to be able to serve families and advocate for humanizing reform within the system. Doula models, then, hold high potential "to open the technocratic system, from the inside, to the possibility of widespread reform" (Davis-Floyd, "Technocratic, Humanistic, Holistic" S10).

Thus, while doula care is on the rise overall, and more hospitals are exploring doula programs for higher risk or under-supported mothers, the position of doulas remains tenuous. The politics of childbirth in the US and the role doula care may play within it is evident, for example, in the media frenzy surrounding a March 2008 *New York Times* article entitled: "And the Doula Makes Four" (Paul). This article reports on a phenomenon called "doula discord," whereby doulas were posited as interfering with the authoritative knowledge of physicians and, at times, even threatening the health and safety of the birthing mother and baby. The article describes a case where a doula was so opposed to medical intervention that she adamantly insisted on "alternatives" to IVs, surgical delivery, and pharmacological pain relief despite the recommendations of the obstetrician and the wishes of the mother. On the surface, this case can be seen as exceptional, an example of the media capitalizing on a rare and extreme occurrence to sell the news. What is enlightening here is that this case gave voice to a fear expressed in some hospitals—that doulas, by virtue of their relationship with the mother who has the right to decline procedures, may undermine the (unquestioned) authority of technocratic providers. Doulas thus become one venue by which bodily knowledge, authoritative medical discourse, and maternity care practices may be contested. This case disrupts the notion of doula as team member and reveals the potential for doula as agitator.

Tension with Homebirth Midwives

Despite the central domains of overlap between midwifery and doula models of care—such as their shared focus on the importance of uninterrupted physiologic birth practices, continuous physical and emotional support, full informed consent, and respect for women's individualized decision-making power—doulas and homebirth midwives may still experience relationships marked by uneasy tension. While most midwives are doulas (especially following intrapartum transfer), most doulas are not midwives. This acknowledgement can produce a wedge, an ambiguity, where friction can be generated between midwives and doulas. We have, for example, heard some midwives question the value of doulas, essentially arguing that doulas enable women to avoid fully rejecting an obstetrician-led, technocratic hospital birth. Because, unlike the midwife, the doula cannot also provide clinical care and, therefore, claim a sphere all her own, doulas may be constructed by midwives as "hospital birth facilitators." In a climate where place of birth has become contentious with very few standing in the middle ground (Cheyney, Burcher, and Vedam), doulas may be perceived as part of the opposition to homebirth. Concurrently, although doulas share care philosophies with midwives, the former may still be seen as ancillary or redundant (at best) or disruptive (at worst) in the homebirth setting. In essence, doulas' liminality is enforced by the fact that they also cannot be fully embraced by homebirth midwives because they facilitate hospital birth and/or claim to advocate for the mother—a role midwives see themselves as fulfilling. This means doulas risk, and sometimes experience, friction with the provider group that, in theory, might be their closest ally.

Homebirth midwives may also claim that doulas are "not resistant enough"—that their models of care, with its majority focus on within-hospital reform, is ultimately a manifestation of systems-correcting, rather than systems-challenging, praxis (Cheyney; Singer). Some midwives argue that, at best, doulas give technocratic care a softer face through their humanizing efforts, and at worst, doulas allow the oppressive system of biomedicine in childbirth to endure. Such midwives contend that doulas essentially help to mystify the unnecessary, even violent (D'Gregorio), practices and outcomes associated with the medical/technocratic model of care. Norman and Rothman have similarly argued that while doulas "have tried to elicit change quietly from within ... the overall result has been an enabling effect. That is, in trying to make quiet waves, doulas ultimately help along the current medicalized system of birth" (280). Doulas—in contrast and in response—claim that they are working to transform the system from the inside out by bringing elements of holistic care into medical spaces. Midwives, however, often claim that doulas may easily become co-opted by this system given their liminal status as at once intimately part of, and marginalized within, hospital-based obstetrics.

The often uneasy relationship between doulas and homebirth midwives can be witnessed in online articles and blog posts that address the working relationships (or lack thereof) between midwives and doulas. For example, a 2014 guest article on the Midwives Alliance blog, entitled "Nine Tips to Help Midwives and Doulas Work Together" (Muza), aimed to address the issues that midwives and doulas encounter in supporting birthing families. Similarly, Citizens for Midwifery ran a thread on their blog and Facebook page in 2011 entitled "Doulas & Homebirth" (Remer). Doulas, parents, and homebirth midwives all weighed in with their perspectives. Midwives often echoed the theme that "every midwife is a doula, but not every doula is a midwife." For example, one midwife wrote, "I have had a couple interviews where a woman has asked if she should have a doula at her homebirth. If someone wants to hire me and a doula, I will not try to talk them out of it. But I see my work as being a doula plus a midwife." In contrast, doulas wrote in about how they view their role in a homebirth: "Providing support for long labours so the midwife can conserve her energy for the important work she might need to do during the actual birth and immediately after. I find myself doula-ing the birth team. Making tea, providing support to the dad, taking pics and of course, supporting the mom as she wishes."

Experiences of mothers who had both—doulas at their home and hospital births—were also present in this thread, demonstrating how doulas can move fluidly to support families across the spectrum:

> *I had the same doula at both my hospital birth and my homebirth and it was well worth it in both cases. At the homebirth she obviously didn't have to function as a warrior/ advocate like she did at the hospital birth, but it was still wonderful to have her there in a supportive role. Having a doula there for mental and physical support provided comfort and assurance, while allowing my husband to be "in the moment" with me while my midwife could focus on the particulars of the labour and delivery themselves.*

This series of remarks ended with these words by article author Molly Remer: "Here's to beautiful, empowering, healthy, fulfilling births for all women, in all settings, with the birth companions of their heart's desire." How, then, can doula and midwifery models of care be strategically aligned to insure greater choice for families across birth settings?

The Power of the Mandorla Space

Doula models of care occupy a mandorla space that is one of uncertain liminality, a transitional space between the two worlds of midwifery/holistic care and medical/technocratic care. This liminal space is not unlike the liminality labouring women experience as they make the physical and psychosocial transition from their pregnant to mothering identities. During these transformative times, women are open to the messages communicated to them by care providers and system models, and they begin to perform the norms that they have received (Butler). The authoritative knowledge valued within medical models of care communicates messages of women's dependency on life-saving technologies and the physicians who deliver them. In contrast, midwifery models of care attempt to communicate messages of empowerment and confidence by constructing women as active subjects and autonomous agents, birthing under the power of their own bodies. Doula models of care sit between these paradigms, bringing elements of one (midwifery care) into the space of another (medical care). Doulas, then, serve as a bridge between these two worlds.

Ultimately, it is within these conceptual and material mandorla spaces that doulas and mothers may engage in forms of resistance that challenge dominant biomedical discourses of childbirth and reveal the potential for transformation. Yet, Norman and Rothman have asked the important question: are doulas "making birth better for women, or just making women feel better about their births?" (262). Ultimately, Norman and Rothman argue that "doulas are in no position to make a revolution" (263), and question whether their positions as "second-class" or even "fourth-class birth workers" (267) ultimately limits their ability to engage in radical change of birthing systems. On the whole, we fundamentally agree that doulas—by the very nature of their liminal position as transitional birthing professionals—are constrained in their potential for resistance. Yet, we see a fissure, an opening, through which doula-attended hospital birth as gendered performance might "slip" (Butler).

As labouring women receive messages of compassion and individualized support through their doulas, they may begin a process of unlearning and relearning, emerging confident in the power of their own bodies, of physiologic birth, and of the role women caring for women can play in Caesarean reduction and healthy outcomes for mother and baby (Cheyney; Everson; Kozhimannil et al.). This may have a profound influence on subsequent birth choices. In this way, hospital-based doula care may unsettle the boundaries of medical models, thus providing a critical opening—a stepping stone—towards midwife-led home and birth centre births as women move through the process of undoing decades of socialization into "birth as medical event" meta-narratives. Indeed, the very presence of a doula may disrupt the "business as usual" routine of hospital procedures, moving obstetricians and nurses (even if only temporarily) into a mandorla space where the presumed wisdom of everyday practice may be questioned. While we both see doula care as valuable in its own right, perhaps if we can also reconceive the liminality of doula care as a potential step toward home and birth centre births, it may be possible to ameliorate some of the friction between midwives and doulas, finding common ground in the power of the mandorla to initiate fundamental reform in childbirth.

CONCLUSION

In conclusion, content analyses of published literature, informed by our ethnographic work as researchers and birth workers, generated five recurring themes that constitute the heart of doula models of care: 1) specialists in the psychosocial needs of childbearing women; 2) support of physiologic birth; 3) provision of individualized, evidence-based support; 4) facilitation of communication and relationship; and 5) continuous companionship. We have argued that doula care occupies a position of liminality, one betwixt and between medical and midwifery models of care. It is in this mandorla space that the potential for systems-wide change occurs as the authoritative knowledge of biomedicine is questioned, and birthing power is placed back into the hands of women. Thus, the strategic alignment of doula and midwifery models of care can be found in the reconceiving of resistance. Rather than constructing resistance discourses against a dichotomous backdrop of home versus hospital, or midwife versus physician—wherein doulas (and families) hover between two worlds, unsure of where their contribution and acceptance lies—we contend that both doula and midwifery models of care can work together to relocate choice and power back to women. Doulas serve as a bridge, holding open the mandorla space where U.S. childbearing models may be negotiated, resisted and, ultimately, transformed. In this way, doula care may enable a widespread shift from hospital-based, medical-dominated systems to one predicated on home and birth centre birth and midwifery-led care for low-risk women. As Michel Odent argues: "If we want to find safe alternatives to obstetrics, we must rediscover midwifery. To rediscover midwifery is the same as giving back childbirth to women." Doulas facilitate such re-discovery through the power of the mandorla space.

WORKS CITED

American College of Nurse Midwives (ACNM), Midwives Alliance of North America (MANA), and the National Association of Certified Professional Midwives (NACPM). "Supporting Healthy and Normal Physiologic Childbirth: A Consensus Statement by the American College of Nurse-Midwives, Midwives Alliance of North America, and the National Association of Certified Professional Midwives." *Journal of Midwifery & Women's Health* 57.5 (2012): 529–532. *NCBI PubMed.* Web. 27 Aug. 2014.

Althabe, Fernando, and José M. Belizán. "Caesarean Section: The Paradox." *Lancet* 368.9546 (2006): 1472–1473. Web. 27 Aug. 2014.

Amnesty International. *Deadly Delivery: The Maternal Health Care Crisis in the USA (One Year Update).* New York: Amnesty International, 2011. Print.

Butler, Judith. *Gender Trouble: Feminism and the Subversion of Identity.* New York: Routledge, 2006. Print.

Childbirth and Postpartum Professional Association (CAPPA). "Position Paper: Evidence-Based Labor Doula Care." Childbirth and Postpartum Professional Association. N.p., 2011. Web. 15 July 2014.

Childbirth and Postpartum Professional Association. "Scope of

Practice: Labor Doula." Childbirth and Postpartum Professional Association. N.p., 2011. Web. 15 July 2014.

Cheyney, Melissa, Paul Burcher, and Saraswathi Vedam. "A Crusade against Home Birth." *Birth* 41.1 (2014): 1-4. Web. 27 Aug. 2014.

Cheyney, Melissa, Courtney Everson, and Paul Burcher. "Home-birth Transfers in the United States: Narratives of Risk, Fear, and Mutual Accommodation." *Qualitative Health Research* 24.4 (2014): 443-456. Web. 27 Aug. 2014.

Cheyney, Melissa J. "Homebirth as Systems-Challenging Praxis: Knowledge, Power, and Intimacy in the Birthplace." *Qualitative Health Research* 18.2 (2008): 254-267. Web. 27 Aug. 2014.

Childbirth Connection. "Doulas and Labor Support | Childbirth Information for Pregnant Women." *Childbirth Connection.* n.p., 2014. Web. 15 July 2014.

Creswell, John W. *Qualitative Inquiry and Research Design: Choosing among Five Approaches.* Thousand Oaks, CA: Sage Publications, 2012. Print.

D'Gregorio, Perez. "Obstetric Violence: A New Legal Term Introduced in Venezuela." *International Journal of Gynecology & Obstetrics* 111.3 (2010): 201-202. Web. 27 Aug. 2014.

Davis-Floyd, R. "The Technocratic, Humanistic, and Holistic Paradigms of Childbirth." *International Journal of Gynaecology and Obstetrics* 75. Suppl 1 (2001): S5-S23. Print.

Davis-Floyd, Robbie E. *Birth as an American Rite of Passage.* Berkeley:University of California Press, 1992. Print.

Declercq, Eugene et al. *Listening to Mothers III: Pregnancy and Birth.* New York: Childbirth Connection, 2013. Print.

DeWalt, Kathleen M. and Billie R. DeWalt. *Participant Observation: A Guide for Fieldworkers.* Lanham, MD: Rowman Altamira, 2010. Print.

Doulas of North America International (DONA). "Position Paper: The Doula's Contribution to Modern Maternity Care." *Doulas of North America International.* N.p., 2012. Web. 15 July 2014.

Emad, Mitra C. "Dreaming the Dark Side of the Body: Pain as Transformation in Three Ethnographic Cases." *Anthropology of Consciousness* 14.2 (2003): 1-26. *Wiley Online Library.* Web. 13 Aug. 2014.

Everson, Courtney L. *"I'm a Mom Too!"—Stigma, Support, &*

Contested Identities among Adolescent Mothers in the United States. Diss., Oregon State University, 2015. Web. 30 Sept. 2015.

Hamilton, Brady E., et al. "Births: Preliminary Data for 2013." *National Vital Statistics Reports* 63.2 (2014): 1-19. Print.

Hays, Danica G., and Anneliese A. Singh. *Qualitative Inquiry in Clinical and Educational Settings*. New York: The Guilford Press, 2011. Print.

Hodnett, Ellen D. et al. "Continuous Support for Women during Childbirth." *The Cochrane Database of Systematic Reviews* 10 (2012): CD003766. Web. 13. Aug. 2014.

International Childbirth Education Association (ICEA). "Position Paper: Physiologic Birth." International Childbirth Education Association. N.p., 2014. Web. 15 July 2014.

International Childbirth Education Association (ICEA). "Position Paper: The Role and Scope of Birth Doula Practice." International Childbirth Education Association. N.p., 2014. Web. 15 July 2014.

Johnson, Robert. *Owning Your Own Shadow: Understanding the Dark Side of the Psyche*. New York: HarperCollins, 1991. Print

Johnson, Christine Barbara, and Robbie Davis-Floyd. "Home to Hospital Transport: Fractured Articulations or Magical Man-dorlas?" *Mainstreaming Midwives: The PoliticsChange*. Ed. Robbie Davis-Floyd and Christine Barbara Johnson. New York: Routledge, 2006. 469-506. Print

Klaus, Marshall H. *Mothering The Mother: How A Doula Can Help You Have A Shorter, Easier, and Healthier Birth*. Reading, Mass: Da Capo Press, 1993. Print.

Kozhimannil, Katy Backes et al. "Potential Benefits of Increased Access to Doula Support During Childbirth." *American Journal of Managed Cared* 20.8 (2014): 1-7. Print.

Lamaze International, Jeanne Green, and Barbara Hotelling. "#3: Bring a Loved One, Friend, or Doula for Continuous Support." *Healthy Birth Practices from Lamaze International*. Washington, DC: Lamaze International. 1-4. Print.

MacDorman, Marian F., T. J. Matthews, and Eugene Declercq. "Trends in out-of-Hospital Births in the United States, 1990-2012." *NCHS Data Brief* 144 (2014): 1–8. Print.

Machizawa, Sayaka and Kayoko Hayashi. "Birthing across Cultures: Toward the Humanization of Childbirth." *Reproductive*

Justice: A Global Concern. Ed. Joan C. Chrisler. Santa Barbara, California: ABC-CLIO, 2012. 231–250. Print.

Morton, Christine and Elayne Clift. *Birth Ambassadors: Doulas and the Re-Emergence of Woman-Supported Birth in America.* Amarillo, TX: Praeclarus Press, 2014. Print.

Muza, Sharon. "Nine Tips To Help Midwives and Doulas Work Together." *Midwives Alliance of North America.* N.p., 2014. Web. 1 June 2014.

Norman, Bari Meltzer and Rothman, Barbara Katz. "The New Arrival: Labor Doulas and the Fragmentation of Midwifery and Caregiving." *Laboring On: Birth in Transition in the United States.* Ed. Wendy Simonds, Barbara Katz Rothman, Bari Meltzer Norman. New York: Routledge, 2007. 251-281. Print.

Paul, Pamela. "And the Doula Makes Four." *NYTimes.com.* New York Times, 2 March 2008. Web. 1 Sept. 2014.

Rayner, Alan David. "Space Cannot Be Cut—Why Self-Identity Naturally Includes Neighbourhood." *Integrative Psychological and Behavioral Science* 45.2 (2011): 161–184. Web. 1 Sept. 2014.

Remer, Molly. "Doulas & Homebirth." *Citizens for Midwifery.* N.p., 2011. Web. 2 June 2014.

Rothman, Barbara Katz. *In Labor: Women and Power in the Birthplace.* New York: W. W. Norton & Co. Incorporated, 1991. Print.

Sandall, Jane, Rona McCandlish, and Debra Bick. "Place of Birth." *Midwifery* 28.5 (2012): 547. Web. 27. Aug. 2014.

Save the Children. *The Urban Disadvantage: State of the World's Mothers 2015.* Fairfield, CT: Save the Children, 2015. Print.

Singer, M. "Beyond the Ivory Tower: Critical Praxis in Medical Anthropology." *Medical Anthropology Quarterly* 9.1 (1995): 80-106; discussion 107-112 passim. Print.

Turner, Victor. *The Forest Symbols: Aspects of Ndembu Ritual.* Ithaca, NY: Cornell University, 1967. 93–111. Print.

Van Gennep, Arnold. *The Rites of Passage.* Chicago, IL: University of Chicago Press, 1960. Print.

Wagner, Marsden. *Born in the USA: How a Broken Maternity System Must Be Fixed to Put Women and Children First.* Berkeley: University of California Press, 2008. Print.

15.
Reimagining the Birthing Body

Reproductive Justice and
New Directions in Doula Care

MONICA BASILE

THE ADVOCACY ROLE OF THE DOULA—its scope and its meaning—is a perennial topic in the world of doula care. Although many doulas see their work as having a long-term transformative effect on hospital protocols and on larger cultural attitudes about birth, the doula's job is most often primarily focused on assisting families on an individual level, and as such, doulas generally tend to view the change that they effect as occurring "one birth at a time."[1] In her research on birth, sociologist Bari Meltzer Norman concludes that doulas are largely "apolitical" and "passive," and that "In trying to make quiet waves, doulas ultimately help along the current medicalized system of birth" (Norman and Rothman 280). Similarly, journalist Jennifer Block wrestles with the idea that doulas may be "perpetuating the very system they are in the business of changing" (160). These assessments raise an important question: to what extent are doulas capable of creating institutional change? Such an inquiry, however, tends to centralize the issue of medicalization as the primary marker of social change related to childbirth. Although this issue is crucial, I argue that the cultural and political impact of doula care extends more broadly. Rather than asking whether doulas can successfully de-medicalize birth, I seek to understand how the doula movement contributes to human rights and social justice through challenging various overlapping axes of inequality, including race, class, gender, and sexuality.

From 2010 to 2012, I conducted ethnographic and survey research across North America with doulas, focusing on how doulas

226

working within a wide variety of settings understand their work.[2] Through this research, and my own experience as a doula for the past twenty years, I have observed that an increasing number of doulas are seeking explicitly to intervene in systemic forms of oppression through providing individualized care to their clients. One doula whom I interviewed, Megan Tate,[3] from Oregon, explained this position succinctly:

> *I appreciate this work because it allows me to cultivate one-on-one connections with people, but I also know that it's bigger than the individuals that I serve. When women reclaim the right to birth on their own terms they might feel more empowered to challenge other forms of oppression and discrimination in their lives.*

Rather than being incapable of, or uninterested in, creating social change, as Norman and Block have suggested, doulas are increasingly working from a political consciousness that perceives birthing choices as part of the spectrum of reproductive rights and as tied to struggles for social justice and human rights.

This perspective is conceptualized by the term "reproductive justice," which the group Forward Together (formerly known as Asian Communities for Reproductive Justice) defines this way:

> Reproductive justice is the complete physical, mental, spiritual, political, economic, and social well-being of women and girls, and will be achieved when women and girls have the economic, social and political power and resources to make healthy decisions about our bodies, sexuality and reproduction for ourselves, our families and our communities in all areas of our lives. (1)

A reproductive justice framework clarifies the connections between birth work and other seemingly unrelated forms of advocacy.[4] The doulas I discuss in this chapter, whom I describe as reproductive justice doulas,[5] are highly attuned to these connections. Their work seeks to address not only the medicalization of childbirth but also larger structural forces that profoundly affect women's lives and their ability to control when and if they have children, how they give birth, the extent to which they are able to provide for their children, and even their children's survival. These doulas are expanding the familiar idea of choice in childbirth in much the same way as feminists of colour have critiqued the pro-choice rhetoric of the abortion rights movement:

> "Choice" implies a marketplace of options in which women's right to determine what happens to their bodies is legally protected, ignoring the fact that for women of color, economic and institutional constraints often restrict their "choices." ...In order to ensure appropriate treatment and access to healthcare and to address the issues of class, race, and gender that affect women of color, a comprehensive human rights-based approach to organizing that accounts for difference is necessary. (Silliman et al. 5, 17)

Although second wave feminist accounts of choice in childbirth have offered insightful analyses of gendered power dynamics in women's health care, most have not adequately attended to the complexities of race and class. The work of contemporary reproductive justice doulas, especially doulas of colour, seeks to address the multilayered disparities in maternity care that are tied to racism and socioeconomic marginalization, such as the far higher rates of mortality for black infants in the U.S.[6]

Research on the effects of doula care has demonstrated clearly and consistently that the presence of a doula improves multiple physical health outcomes (Hodnett et al.). However, medical anthropologists have argued that health is not only physical but also inherently social and political; it is a dynamic process rather than a static, quantifiable physical state. Margaret Lock and Nancy Scheper-Hughes assert that there are "three bodies" that merit analytical attention: the individual body; the social body, in which the body functions symbolically; and the body politic, encompassing the social "regulation, surveillance, and control of bodies (individual and collective) in reproduction and sexuality, work, leisure, and sickness" (7-8). I argue that doulas are increasingly attending to the social body and the body politic through their

228

work with the individual body. I observe that doulas are expanding the traditional model of one-on-one birth care through innovative projects that seek to empower people in multiple facets of their lives, beyond the birthing room. In this chapter, I outline several emerging doula models and identities: community-based doulas, prison doulas, full-spectrum doulas, and radical doulas. I argue that these new directions in doula care are driving productive and vital connections between birthing rights advocacy and a broad-based reproductive justice approach, linking reproductive health care and social justice.

COMMUNITY-BASED DOULAS

Community-based doulas (CBDs), in contrast to private doulas, practise within programs that are designed to "serve communities that have been self-defined as underserved" (Abramson 31). CBDs are usually members of the same racial, ethnic, and/or socioeconomic background as the people whom they serve, and are often already leaders within those communities. The organization Health Connect One is at the forefront of developing the CBD model, assisting communities in creating CBD programs, and securing funding for them. Currently, Health Connect One reports that there are fifty-two community-based doula programs operating in eighteen states, and forty-six more are in development, all serving a diverse range of communities (Health Connect One).

The CBD model is derived from the community health worker approach, wherein the community health worker is an "insider who is employed in a formal role that transforms her community" (Abramson 23). The Chicago Doula Project, which began its pilot project in 1996, is the forerunner of many of the community-based doula programs that currently operate. Its success has led to the development of teams of trainers and consultants who partner with interested communities and assist them in establishing their own doula programs. The education of doulas in the Chicago Health Connection community-based doula program is based on a Freirean popular education model and has been characterized as a process "by which people are supported in recognizing their own power to take action in their lives" (Abramson 19). Trainers in this program explain that "training for change begins with personal awareness and connects to a more political analysis or 'critical consciousness'" (Abramson 19). The community-based doulas in my study exemplify this type of consciousness in the ways in which they describe the larger impact of their work. For example, Ellen Ridley, a doula who works with a community-based program in Illinois, is attentive to the reverberations of her work into the community itself:

> *Especially working with underprivileged teens like I do, a lot of what we do deals with making sure that young mothers are supported and bond with their babies in the hope that cycles of abuse and neglect that may have ravaged certain neighborhoods or families might come to an end. We hope for good beginnings with each baby.*

For Ellen, supporting individual women is akin to supporting an entire neighbourhood. Some of the community-based doulas in my study described the larger effects of their work as occurring generationally. Josefina Cavazos, a doula who works with a program serving indigenous women in Los Angeles, said, "I hope my work influences the next seven generations. I hope that my work influences my daughters and future granddaughters to believe in and want natural childbirth." Others also made connections between the power of birth in one's body and one's political power. Jessica Lomas, who works with a doula collective in Washington, said:

> *It's powerful to feel like you are creating change in your own body. If you feel capable in your own skin of growing and birthing and raising a child, then how does that affect our involvement in other social justice issues? Powerfully! I think it's what Obama said: We can do it! It's gonna be tough, but it's not about instant gratification.*

Whereas the idea of one birth at a time reinforces the individuality of birth experiences—one mother, one family, one baby—the attitude toward social change described by many community-based doulas is more grounded in the effects of a birth experience on the families and communities that the birthing mother and her child are connected to. This perspective reflects the idea that a doula's involvement has the power to strengthen those connections and inspire people to pass certain values, such as political involvement, down to their children.

PRISON DOULAS: "BRINGING BACK A SENSE OF HOME"

At the time of my research, there were three prison doula projects in the United States: the Birth Attendants in Olympia, Washington (founded in 2002); the Prison Birth Project in Amherst, Massachusetts (founded in 2008); and the Isis Rising Prison doula program in Minneapolis, Minnesota (founded in 2012). The forerunner to these programs in the U.S. is London, England's Birth Companions program, which started in 1996. Each of these prison doula programs integrates three main components: doulas and childbirth educators provide classes and support groups to pregnant women and mothers in prison; they provide direct support during labour and birth; and they undertake networking, collaborations with other organizations, and community awareness related to incarcerated mothers' issues. For example, the Birth Attendants program holds a reproductive justice book club in the community to raise awareness about incarcerated mothers.[7]

I conducted face-to-face interviews with Aliyah Jones, Alex Snyder, and Cassidy Wolfson, three of the Birth Attendants doulas in Olympia. As members of the first such program in the U.S., they detailed the ways in which their work is unique in the fields of both doula work and prison work. While private doulas focus their efforts on the labor and birth experience, prison doulas place more of their attention on prenatal and postpartum support. Because incarcerated women have so many unique and unmet needs during pregnancy and the postpartum period, the Birth Attendants doulas' work is much more focused on childbirth education, community building, and postpartum assistance. Because infants are routinely separated from their incarcerated mothers,[8] postpartum support for incarcerated women cannot revolve around everyday parenting tasks such as feeding, diapering, and bathing but instead focuses on acknowledging the complex feelings that accompany parental separation and perhaps finding ways to create bonds with a child who is not currently in the mother's care.

Like the community-based doulas in Chicago, the Birth Attendants use a popular education approach. Aliyah described their group structure:

> We don't believe in having a structured curriculum—our classes follow a popular education model. What are someone's needs right now? What happened at their last prenatal appointment? We have lots of books and videos for them to check out. Things are always changing. Depending on who comes, the topic changes. This works really well. It helps us to be sharpened in our skills, and we learn too. If we don't know an answer, we'll look at our resources together to try to figure it out.

By learning with and from the women in prison, these doulas create relationships that are non-hierarchical, and this is a core value shared by the Birth Attendants doulas. The Birth Attendants are also unique in comparison with other prison workers in that they are not affiliated with religious or other institutions or organizations. Aliyah emphasized the unconditional support their organization offers:

> We are special in that we're not Christian, like so many other groups that come into the prisons. We're not bringing in Bibles. The language used to describe the people is "offenders" and "inmates." We don't ever ask what they've done. If someone wants a cesarean, that's their choice. We just support them. We're not trying to convert anybody. Most other groups are religiously affiliated, but we're here to advocate and be conduits of information. Every person should be supported wherever they're at, from cesarean section to unassisted childbirth. People need access to information.

For the Birth Attendants, a non-judgmental attitude toward a person's criminal background is parallel to a non-judgmental attitude toward the birth method and outcome. Aliyah is "not trying to convert" anyone, either in terms of religion, or in terms of birth method. Because the women prison doulas serve are already in a vulnerable place and subject to the most coercive of institutional constraints, it becomes even more important for prison doulas to afford them as much choice as possible about their birth experiences.

The Birth Attendants also witness the powerful ways in which the power structures of the prison intersect with those in the hospital. Cassidy described what it is like to support an incarcerated woman during labour and delivery:

> *Advocating for women in prison is the hardest. People [working at the hospital] have preconceived notions, and sometimes assumptions that people are less educated. [Hospital staff] are frustrated when a client [from the prison] comes in with a birth plan. The idea is: what makes you think you have the right? They're looked at as people who shouldn't be having a baby.*

This observation mirrors those of many doulas around the country who work with women who may be socially coded as not "legitimate mothers" (Solinger).

Like community-based doulas, the Birth Attendants see their work not so much as working to make small changes one birth at a time but as breaking down barriers and creating connections. Alex said:

> *Prison is an energy force that thrives on breaking down community. It thrives on divisions, like racism. We are not affiliated with anyone, and that breaks down barriers, creates community on the inside. There's not always an opportunity for people from minimum and maximum security to meet. There's not that ability to talk with your sister. We're bringing it back to the simplicity of "we're human," bringing back a sense of home.*

Prison doulas, in serving physically and socially marginalized people, are intervening powerfully in the structures upholding that marginalization, simply by asserting and affirming the basic humanity of the incarcerated.

FULL-SPECTRUM DOULAS

The term "full-spectrum doula" is used to describe a person who offers not only labour and birth support but also support through a wide range of reproductive experiences, including abortion, adoption (for both birth and adoptive parents), miscarriage, and stillbirth. In 2007, doulas Mary Mahoney and Lauren Mitchell began the Abortion Doula Project in New York City, with the intention of providing information, emotional support, relaxation techniques, and physical support to people choosing to terminate pregnancies. As they became more involved in this work, they found that the needs of their clients were larger than anticipated, and their organization, now simply called the Doula Project, now contracts with several clinics and organizations in New York City to provide full-spectrum doula services.[9]

Because of the politicization of abortion, the emotional context of the abortion experience has been politicized as well; anti-abortion advocates make claims about its traumatic effects, and abortion rights advocates argue that most women feel relieved about their choice to terminate an unwanted pregnancy. The idea of supporting a person through the abortion experience, therefore, is potentially off-putting to some supporters of abortion rights, even though abortion doulas identify across the board as pro-choice. Mary Mahoney, one of the founders of the Doula Project, explains her response to this dilemma in an interview on the Exhale blog:

> Some people in the reproductive health and rights movement have asked us, why do you assume women having abortions need emotional support? In the beginning, that question scared me. I thought, is that what our project is doing? Are we setting the movement back in some way by thinking that this is an emotional time for a woman? What I've learned is that everyone experiences abortion, and pregnancy for that matter, differently…. So I've stopped

making generalizations or trying to predict how a woman will react before, during, or after her abortion because each person's life looks different, even within a shared physical experience. And I stopped being scared of the movement when I started getting to know the individual having the abortion. Nearly all of the individuals we've encountered in the clinic have benefited from doula support, whether on an emotional (which can have a variety of meanings), physical, or informational level. (Mahoney Interview)

By refusing to make abortion doula work fit neatly and completely into pro-choice arguments about the emotions surrounding abortion, Mahoney makes room for people's real life experiences to exceed the heightened rhetoric on either side of the abortion debate.

The founders of the Doula Project identified the need for adoption doula services after hearing stories from allied professionals working in an adoption agency. In an online article entitled "The Doula Movement: Making the Radical a Reality by Trusting Pregnant Women," Mahoney describes learning about "nurses and doctors not respecting the [birth] mothers' wishes to have the baby taken out of the room following the birth, or just the opposite, nurses not letting the mothers hold or breastfeed their newborns since they were choosing not to parent." Adoption doulas may provide support to both birth parents and adoptive parents. They typically offer private, adoption-specific childbirth education; postpartum support that includes assistance and support for various choices regarding breastfeeding and pumping; help in escorting the birth mother home from the hospital if she is alone; referral to other counselling or support resources as needed; and uninterrupted labour support and assistance in making birth plans. They also may serve adoptive families by offering childbirth education specific to the needs of adopting families and help with bonding, infant feeding choices, and general newborn care.

Full-spectrum doulas also provide support during pregnancy loss. Even if a doula sets out to work solely as a birth doula she will likely, at some point, be called on to support someone who has had a miscarriage or stillbirth. In addition to grief support and other forms of emotional support, those experiencing pregnancy losses face bodily experiences and medical treatment options that can be difficult to navigate without the benefit of informational support. As anthropologist Linda Layne argues, pregnancy loss is rendered all but invisible within the mainstream natural child-birth movement, with its emphasis on joyful, ecstatic depictions of birth. Layne calls for a woman-centred and accessible model of care for those experiencing loss, and her recommendations closely mirror the support doulas are increasingly providing. Full-spectrum doulas are in a powerful position to challenge the erasure of pregnancy loss within the childbirth movement. Full-spectrum doulas recognize that the needs of pregnant women go far beyond and are far more complicated than the politically opposing poles of pro- and anti-choice.

RADICAL DOULAS

A growing number of doulas are identifying themselves as radical doulas.[10] Radical doulas tend to espouse an intersectional politics that embraces a multiplicity of identity, and a commitment to making doula care more accessible to marginalized communities. These goals are connected in that they represent a challenge to dominant conceptions of the embodiment of both "good" mothers and "good" doulas (white, middle class, cisgender female, part-nered, heterosexual, English speaking, etc.). The vast majority of doulas in my study, whether or not they were part of programs that specifically reach out to underserved people, have provided care to clients with challenges related to structural inequalities. More than half of the doulas in my survey report having assisted single parents, teen parents, low-income parents, and abuse survivors. Almost half of the doulas in my study have assisted immigrants or refugees, English language learners, LGBTQ people, or current or former drug users.[11] It is often through these experiences that doulas become "radicalized." Many doulas in my study related accounts about the differential treatment of clients. Jane Halliday in Wisconsin said:

Most striking was the difference in treatment in the hospitals and by nurses for my clients who were women of color, low

income or teenage—many fitting into all of these categories.
I have seen RNs say things to them that are so hurtful and
discouraging and would never be said to a private client
who was white, well educated, and over twenty-five.

Kimberly Greenlee in Washington, DC, echoed this sentiment, stating, "L&D nurses are sometimes pretty rude to teen moms. I hear comments like, 'you should have thought of how painful it was going to be before you went and got pregnant!'" And Norma Jameson in Connecticut observed, "In caring for same sex couples, I find that there are more barriers to communication in the hospital. The non-pregnant mother is not seen as a parent by some caregivers." In situations like these, in advocating for the client, the doula is advocating not only for humanizing a particular birth experience but also for the humane treatment of a marginalized population. Through these types of experiences, doulas are becoming increasingly attuned to a reproductive justice model as they witness the intersection of autonomy in birth with LGBT rights, abortion rights, prisoners' rights, teen parents' rights, and economic and racial justice.

Many doulas whom I surveyed indicated that they feel especially drawn to expanding access to doula care, and for many of them, this is tied to their own racial, ethnic, sexual, gender, or political identities. For instance, Joanna Tilley, in Minnesota shared:

[Being a radical doula] means I practice as an OUT lesbian
in my community. It means I work with the choice commu-
nity to bring women's reproductive freedom to the clinic as
well as the birth room. It means I push women to think for
themselves and take their birth to a spiritual level, make it
a life altering experience. It means I encourage women to
let go of shame about their bodies, their sex, their fears.

For Joanna, her own visibility as a lesbian doula and the public presentation of pro-choice, feminist politics is a key part of the service that she provides.

Although the doula profession is made up mostly of cisgender women, there are male, transgender, gender nonconforming, and

genderqueer doulas practicing today. Four doulas in my study identified themselves as male, and one as genderqueer. Jason Epstein,
one of male doulas in my study, also experiences his identity as a
radical quality on multiple levels:

> *I feel like it is radical to really be willing to support people
> in birth in the way that is truly safe and comfortable for
> them. I am also queer socialized and sex positive which
> feels important for many people in birth. Although I don't
> think it should be, apparently being a male doula is radical.
> I also offer abortion doula support.*

Jason indicated, as did many other survey respondents, that there
are childbearing families who do not seek doula services from
more heteronormative doulas because it does not feel "truly safe
and comfortable," and who are actively seeking care from doulas
who are "queer socialized and sex positive." Like doulas working
in community-based programs, many radical doulas recognize the
importance and safety of shared identities between doula and client.

For many of the reproductive justice doulas in my survey, it has
also become important to use gender-neutral language to refer to
pregnant people. Laurel Ripple Carpenter draws attention to the
need for greater gender inclusivity among birthworkers in an article
in *SQUAT Birth Journal*. She reminds the reader that "We are not
all women" and that "There are doulas and midwives across the
whole spectrum of gender diversity who are challenging the notion
that midwifery is women's work" (28). The use of gender-neutral
language, and the recognition of transgender and gender variant
experiences of parenthood, de-links gender from pregnancy and
childbirth—experiences that are generally considered quintessen-
tially female. As such, this move among some doulas represents a
radical re-thinking of the meaning of sex and gender and a profound
challenge to an essentialist, binary gender system.

The need for greater racial diversity within the doula community—and for greater understanding of issues of racism and privilege
as they relate to birthing politics and practices—is also a priority
of many self-identified radical doulas. It was clear in my research
that radical doulas actively sought training that addresses racism

and cultural competence, such as that offered by the International Center for Traditional Childbearing (ICTC). Known as the Full Circle Doula program, the ICTC doula training model "creates leaders to advocate the normalcy of birth, reduce infant mortality, support breastfeeding and develop entrepreneur skills to combat poverty" (ICTC *Doula Training* 1). Created by Shafia Monroe in 2002, ICTC's doula program has now trained over 500 doulas, with 85 percent being women of colour (ICTC *History*). Doulas of North America—or DONA, the largest doula training organization—is also actively working to increase racial diversity among its members, trainers, and leaders.

LOOKING FORWARD

Although the majority of the doulas whom I surveyed are serving a wide range of people with a variety of needs, mainstream doula training still reflects an orientation toward working with a rather narrow range of families. Most doulas in my study said that they were not prepared by their training for the advocacy circumstances they have encountered. Bearing witness to the overlapping forces of social injustice and birthing injustice was identified as a significant source of stress for many doulas, especially since so few doulas felt adequately prepared to effectively advocate in these situations. My study showed that doulas all around the country are struggling with how to advocate for people who often have very complex sets of needs, and if they are not part of a community-based program, they are doing so with little formalized help. As doulas increasingly come up against issues of reproductive justice, new opportunities for awareness-raising, community formation, and advocacy are emerging.

In addition to cultural competency, the concept of structural competency in health care settings is beginning to be more widely recognized among birthworkers, paving the way for increased attention to structural competency in doula training.[12] A growing attention to diversity is reflected in DONA's member publication, *The International Doula*, which recently has included an article about working with adolescents, a profile of a hospital-based doula group working with HIV positive mothers, and the "Ask

Penny Simkin" column translated into Spanish. Most recently, *The International Doula* has featured an extensive interview with Sherry Payne, founder of the organization Uzazi Village, whose mission is to decrease black infant mortality and racially-based health inequities. In the interview, Payne speaks powerfully about racial disparities in maternal and child health, the importance of the work of doulas of colour, and some of the challenges and barriers that they face within the doula community.

Public funding on both a state and federal level has increased access to doula care. In 2012, the Oregon state legislature passed a bill that required the Oregon Health Authority to investigate how doulas and other community health workers could improve birth outcomes for the state's underserved families. The investigation reported that doula care is an effective way to decrease health inequities, and it led to legislation incorporating doulas into the Oregon Health Plan, making them eligible for reimbursement by Medicaid and Medicare. In 2013, Minnesota followed suit and became the second state in the U.S. with legislation requiring Medicaid payment for doula services.

Although these legislative breakthroughs have expanded access to doulas in these states, some difficulties have arisen in the implementation of this legislation. The 2015 executive summary evaluating the Minnesota program lists several challenges, including low reimbursement rates for doulas. Additionally, since doulas are non-licensed care providers, they must provide services under the supervision of a licensed clinician in order to be reimbursed. This presents further structural difficulties for doulas seeking Medicaid coverage (Kozhimannil et al. i). The Minnesota summary lays out a detailed set of concerns and potential solutions, and is an important document that can assist doulas and advocates in Minnesota and in other states as they work toward similar legislation.

Federal funding for community-based doula programs has also increased with the passage of the Affordable Care Act in 2010, which provides for the expansion of Community Health Centers and Community Based Doula (CBD) programs. The 2014 Health Connect One report—*The Perinatal Revolution,* supported jointly by the U.S. Health Resources and Services Administration (HRSA) and the Centers for Disease Control and Prevention (CDC)—provides a comprehensive exploration of the achievements of the community-based doula model, implications for health policy, and recommendations for the further development and integration of this model into U.S. health systems. Echoing earlier research on CBD programs, the report lists extensive social and economic benefits associated with a reduction of premature and Caesarean births, an increase in breastfeeding duration, and an increased use of preventive health care services (27-32). The report emphasizes that the Affordable Care Act provides an important opportunity for further integrating CBD programs into existing Community Health Centers, and recommends providing CBD funding to each federally funded Community Health Center. The implications for long-term sustainability of CBD programs is also an important focus of the report, which recommends the promotion of public and private funding partnerships and further emphasizes that "while discretionary, grant-funded programs are important, integration of community-based doula programs with mandatory programs may lend itself to a more long-term solution" (42). As this report demonstrates, if CBDs are to be optimally integrated into the U.S. health care workforce, funding for the multilayered services that they provide needs to be secure.

It is clear that a shift is taking place in the ways that doula care is being accessed and understood. *The Perinatal Revolution* report concludes by describing a changing attitude toward social determinants of health:

> There is a growing understanding that investments in pre- and inter-conceptional, pregnancy, birth and early childhood support are essential for the health of our population and economy.... The community-based doula is a role that makes use of social capital and of the power of relationships to improve health and development in communities facing huge challenges. The Community-Based Doula Program integrates community experience with systems of care at a powerful moment in the life of families. (48)

This is also a powerful moment for maternal-child health policy advocates and childbirth reformers to make a difference by turning their attention to doulas and the vital role that they play in both individual and community health. Institutional and community support are essential for the continued development of doula projects that are attuned to addressing health disparities and social injustice.

Reproductive justice doulas—including community-based doulas, prison doulas, full-spectrum doulas, and radical doulas—are forging new pathways to bring together social justice activism and birthwork. They are incorporating an intersectional approach to doula care by recognizing that the continuum of reproductive experiences are shaped by structures of privilege and oppression, and they are asserting everyone's right to competent support within those experiences and structures. They are shifting the questions childbirth reformers raise beyond the single issue of medicalization and toward equality, access, and justice, thereby changing the frame through which the effects of medicalization are understood. By centring new priorities and expanding the scope of services offered, reproductive justice doulas are finding connections among contradictions and challenging individualistic and binary ways of thinking about bodies and reproductive issues. As doulas increasingly connect their work to other forms of social justice advocacy, they are in a powerful position from which to redefine the scope of childbirth reform in the U.S. in the twenty-first century.

ENDNOTES

[1]This is a recurring phrase among doulas. It is also noted by sociologist Christine Morton in her research on doula practice, which outlines the complex interactions and negotiations doulas undertake in the hospital setting.

[2]My research focused on how doulas take action to bring about changes in the culture and experience of pregnancy and birth, and the goals and effects birthworkers ascribe to their work, both as activists and professionals. I used face-to-face interviews and online surveys, gathered after approval from the Institutional Review Board (IRB# 200903769). I also participated in two major conferences for birthworkers and activists: National Advocates for Pregnant

Women in 2007, and the Midwives Alliance of North America regional conference in 2009. I conducted face-to-face interviews with 15 doulas, and 156 doulas completed my survey, comprising doulas from 40 states and five Canadian provinces. The average age of survey respondents was 32 years old (oldest 68, youngest 20). The vast majority of survey respondents identified as female, four identified as male, and one as genderqueer. I asked respondents to identify their race/ethnicity as an open-ended question: 84 percent of respondents identified as white; 11 percent as black; 3 percent as Native American/American Indian; 2 percent as Hispanic/Latina; 1 percent each as Jewish, white/Hispanic, Asian/Pacific Islander, Afro-Latina, and biracial/mixed-race. The vast majority of survey respondents, 94 percent, had some college education, and 68 percent had college degrees. For more information, see Basile, "*Reproductive Justice.*"

[3] All names of interviewees in this chapter are pseudonyms.

[4] For more about the development of reproductive justice, see Zakiya Luna and Kristin Luker.

[5] This is my own theoretical framing, although some individual doulas do refer to themselves in this way.

[6] In 2009, low birth weight was at seven percent for white infants, and almost 14 percent for black infants (Martin 12). The infant mortality rate in 2007 for white babies was 5.6/1000 births and 13.3/1000 for black babies (Mathews 3).

[7] The number of women incarcerated in the U.S. has risen by 400 percent since the introduction of federal mandatory sentencing for drug offences in the 1980s, and the percentage of women incarcerated for drug offenses is now greater than that of males (Sabol et al.). About five percent of women entering state prisons are pregnant, and six percent of women in jails are pregnant. Most women in prison are survivors of sexual and physical abuse, and women of colour are disproportionately imprisoned, comprising nearly two-thirds of all women held in federal, state, and local jails and prisons (Schroeder and Bell 54). The Rebecca Project, which investigates policies affecting incarcerated mothers and their children, reports that pregnant women lack quality prenatal care (National Women's Law Center 10). In 2008, the Federal Bureau of Prisons ended the routine shackling of pregnant inmates in fed-

eral correctional facilities. State governments have begun to follow suit, but only a handful of states have laws prohibiting shackling during labour. (National Women's Law Center 2010:11).

[8]This is typically the case, although some prisons do have nursery programs. The prison in Olympia does have such a program, but women must meet tightly defined criteria to be eligible.

[9]At this time, there are full-spectrum doula services in many cities across the country, including Seattle, Atlanta, Chicago, Boston, Philadelphia, and Asheville, North Carolina (*Radical Doula,* "Volunteer Programs").

[10]Miriam Zoila Perez writes the Radical Doula blog, authored the 2012 *Radical Doula Guide,* and her name is now associated with the radical doula movement. Although this designation now resonates with many, "radical doula" is still an emerging identity. Many doulas in my study expressed confusion or ambivalence about what this might mean. Some explicitly disavow the term because they dislike the connotation of a "fringe and extreme activist" or interpret it as referring to a doula who practices outside the widely accepted scope of practice.

[11]Fewer doulas have assisted clients who are homeless, incarcerated, disabled, planning to release a baby for adoption or terminate a pregnancy, but the vast majority of doulas indicated that they would be willing to assist women in any of those categories. Of course, doulas or care providers may also fall into any of the above listed categories, as well.

[12]See, for example, Metzl and Hansen, who describe structural competency as "a shift in medical education away from pedagogic approaches to stigma and inequalities that emphasize cross-cultural understandings of individual patients, toward attention to forces that influence health outcomes at levels above individual interactions" (126).

WORKS CITED

Abramson, Rachel, Ginger Breedlove, and Beth Isaacs. *The Community-Based Doula: Supporting Families Before, During, and After Childbirth.* Washington, DC: Zero to Three Press, 2006. Print.

Asian Communities for Reproductive Justice. *A New Vision for Advancing Our Movement for Reproductive Health, Reproductive Rights, and Reproductive Justice.* Oakland, CA: Forward Together, 2005. Pdf.

Basile, Monica. *Reproductive Justice and Childbirth Reform: Doulas as Agents of Social Change.* Diss., University of Iowa, 2012.

Block, Jennifer. *Pushed: The Painful Truth About Childbirth and Modern Maternity Care.* Cambridge, MA: Da Capo Press, 2007. Print.

Carpenter, Laurel Ripple. "We are Not All Women: Midwives, Doulas, and the Gender of Birth Work." *SQUAT Birth Journal* (Summer 2011): 28-29. Print.

Health Connect One. *Programs and Training: Community-Based Doula Program Replication.* Health Connect One, 2014. Web. 12 Nov. 2015.

Health Connect One. *The Perinatal Revolution.* Health Connect One, 2014. Web. 12 Nov. 2015. Pdf.

Hodnett, Ellen D. et al. "Continuous Support for Women during Childbirth." *The Cochrane Database of Systematic Reviews* 10 (2012): CD003766. *NCBI PubMed.* Web. 12 Nov. 2015.

International Center for Traditional Childbearing (ICTC). *ICTC History.* ICTC, 2015. Web. 12 Nov. 2015.

International Center for Traditional Childbearing (ICTC). *The ICTC Doula Training Program.* ICTC, n.d. Web. 12 Nov 2015. Pdf.

Kozhimannil, Katy B., Carrie A. Vogelsang, and Rachel R. Hardeman. *Medicaid Coverage of Doulas in Minnesota: Preliminary Findings from the First Year: Interim Report to the Minnesota Department of Public Services.* Everyday Miracles, July 2015. Web. 12 Nov. 2015. Pdf.

Layne, Linda. *Motherhood Lost: A Feminist Account of Pregnancy Loss in America.* New York: Routledge, 2002. Print.

Lock, Margaret and Nancy Scheper-Hughes. "The Mindful Body: A Prolegomenon to Future Work in Medical Anthropology." *Medical Anthropology Quarterly* New Series 1.1 (1987): 6-41. Print.

Luna, Zakiya and Kristin Luker. "Reproductive Justice." *Annual Review of Law and Social Science* 9 (2013): 327–52. Print.

Mahoney, Mary. "Interview with Mary Mahoney of the Doula

Project." Interview by Aspen Baker. *Exhale*. 8 Mar. 2010. Web. 12 Nov. 2015.

Mahoney, Mary. "The Doula Movement: Making the Radical a Reality by Trusting Pregnant Women." *RH Reality Check*. n.p, 27 Jan. 2010. Web. 20 Aug. 2014.

Metzl, Jonathan M. and Helena Hansen. "Structural Competency: Theorizing a New Medical Engagement with Stigma and Inequality." *Social Science & Medicine* 103 (2013): 126-133. Print.

Morton, Christine and Elayne Clift. *Birth Ambassadors: Doulas and the Re-Emergence of Woman-Supported Birth in America*. Amarillo, TX: Praeclarus Press, 2014. Print.

Nelson, Jennifer. *Women of Color and the Reproductive Rights Movement*. New York: New York University Press, 2003. Print.

Perez, Miriam. *The Radical Doula Guide: A Political Primer for Full Spectrum Pregnancy and Childbirth Support*. Self-published, 2012. Print.

Perez, Miriam. *Radical Doula Blog: Volunteer Programs*. N.p, n.d. Web. 11 Nov. 2015.

Rebecca Project for Human Rights. *Mothers Behind Bars: A State-by-State Report Card and Analysis of Federal Policies on Conditions of Confinement for Pregnant and Parenting Women and the Effect on Their Children*. Washington, DC: National Women's Law Center, 2012. Pdf.

Sabol, William J., Heather C. West and Matthew Cooper. *Bureau of Justice Statistics Bulletin: Prisoners in 2008*. U.S. Department of Justice, Dec. 2009. Web. 30 June 2010. Pdf.

Schroeder, Carole and Janice Bell. "Doula Birth Support for Incarcerated Pregnant Women." *Public Health Nursing* 22.1 (2005): 53-58. Print.

Silliman, Jael, Marlene Gerber Fried, Loretta Ross, and Elena Gutierrez. *Undivided Rights: Women of Color Organize for Reproductive Justice*. Cambridge, MA: South End Press, 2004. Print.

Simonds, Wendy, Barbara Katz Rothman, and Bari Meltzer Norman. *Laboring On: Birth in Transition in the United States*. New York: Routledge, 2007. Print.

Solinger, Rickie. *Pregnancy and Power: A Short History of Reproductive Politics in America*. New York: New York University Press, 2005. Print.

Contributor Notes

Monica Basile holds a PhD in gender, women's, and sexuality studies. Her 2012 dissertation, *Reproductive Justice and Childbirth Reform: Doulas as Agents of Social Change,* explores the intersections of doula work and reproductive justice. She is also a certified professional midwife, certified doula, and childbirth educator, and has been an activist and birth worker for the past twenty years.

Alison Bastien is an anthropologist, childbirth educator, and retired certified professional midwife in homebirth practice. She dedicates her time now to teaching midwifery and natural medicine, doing consultations in women's health issues, and supervising the herbal workshop and store where her family sells herbal products in central Mexico.

Angela N. Castañeda, PhD, CD (DONA) is associate professor and Edward Myers Dolan professor of anthropology at DePauw University. Her research in Brazil, Mexico, and the U.S. explores questions on religion, ritual, expressive culture, and the cultural politics of reproduction, birth, and motherhood. She is a practising birth and postpartum doula, as well as a volunteer Spanish childbirth educator in Bloomington, Indiana, where she lives with her family.

Melissa Cheyney, PhD, CPM, LDM, is an associate professor of medical anthropology and reproductive biology in the Anthropology Program at Oregon State University in Corvallis, Oregon.

She is also a certified professional midwife, licensed in the state of Oregon, the chair of the MANA Division of Research, and the director of the OSU Reproductive Health Laboratory.

Megan Davidson, PhD, is a Brooklyn, New York-based labour and postpartum doula, a childbirth educator, and a breastfeeding counselor who has attended over four hundred births and assisted over a thousand families in the immediate postpartum period. Also an anthropologist, Megan is interested in the social construction of sexed bodies and gender identities, cultural and biological under-standings of reproduction and birth, the politics of motherhood, activism, and social change.

Robbie Davis-Floyd, PhD, senior research fellow, Department of Anthropology, University of Texas, Austin, and fellow of the Society for Applied Anthropology, is a world-renowned medical anthro-pologist, international speaker and researcher in transformational models in childbirth, midwifery, and obstetrics. She is author of over eighty articles and of *Birth As an American Rite of Passage* (1992, 2004), co-author of *From Doctor to Healer: The Trans-formative Journey* (1998) and *The Power of Ritual* (forthcoming 2016), and lead editor of ten collections, the latest of which is *Birth Models That Work* (2009), which highlights optimal models of birth care around the world. Her current research project studies the paradigm shifts of holistic obstetricians. Robbie serves as edi-tor for the *International MotherBaby Childbirth Initiative* (www. imbci.org) and senior advisor to the Council on Anthropology and Reproduction. Most of her published articles are freely available on her website: www.davis-floyd.com.

Courtney Everson, PhD, is a biocultural medical anthropologist and the graduate dean at the Midwives College of Utah in Salt Lake City, Utah. She is also the director of Research Education for the MANA Division of Research; the vice president of the Oregon Doula Association; a birth doula practitioner; and serves on the Boards of Directors for the Australasian Professional Doula Regulatory Association and Oregon Doula Connection. Dr. Everson's research addresses doula and midwifery care, as mother-centered care models, for reducing health inequities and improving maternal-infant well-being, with a focus on pregnant and parenting adolescents.

Nicole C. Gallicchio is a medical anthropologist whose doctoral dissertation at the University of Chicago explores the processes by which birth doulas learn to provide empowered, ethical care through their navigation of the complex political, moral, and psychosocial landscapes of contemporary American childbirth. She currently lives and works in Oslo, where she is exploring Norwegian socialized medical support for reproductive health.

Amy L. Gilliland, PhD, BDT (DONA), CD (DONA), CSE (AASECT), researches and teaches about doula labour support, women's sexual experiences, and the psychological needs of mothers and fathers during the birth experience. She is an AASECT certified sexuality educator, a member of the psychology faculty at Madison College, and one of the first DONA International birth doula trainers. Dr. Gilliland's research has been published in *JOGNN*, *Midwifery*, *Journal of Perinatal Education*, *Sexuality and Culture*, and the *Wisconsin Medical Journal*.

Maria E. Hamilton Abegunde, PhD, is an egungun (ancestral) priest in the Yoruba Orisa tradition and Reiki master. As a Black studies scholar, she explores the links between unresolved ancestral emotions, urban violence, and illness. She is a birth and postpartum doula.

Nicole Heidbreder is a labour and delivery nurse at George Washington University Hospital. She is also a birth doula trainer through DONA International and a childbirth educator and lactation counselor. Nicole lives and works in Washington, DC. More information can be found here: www.gracefulfusion.com.

Marisha L. Humphries, PhD, is an associate professor in the Department of Educational Psychology and a licensed clinical psychologist. Her research seeks to develop an integrated approach to studying African-American children's normative and prosocial development, and utilizing this basic research to create culturally and developmentally appropriate school-based behaviour promotion programs.

Jacqueline Kelleher has been supporting growing families since 1996 as a birth and postpartum doula, childbirth educator, lactation counselor, doula trainer-mentor, and community volunteer. She served as the director of Postpartum Services for DONA International and continues as a DONA postpartum doula mentor. She is the author of *Nurturing The Family: The Guide for Postpartum Doulas*.

Jon Korfmacher, PhD, is an Associate Professor at Erikson Institute, a graduate school in child development in Chicago, Illinois. His research examines the implementation and outcome of early childhood interventions, parent engagement as well as policies and practices in early childhood mental health, with an emphasis on workforce training and development.

Sarah Lewin, LMSW, is a labour doula working in New York City. She received her Masters in Social Work at New York University and attended The Women's Therapy Centre Institute's psychoanalytic training, studying relationships to food and body from a feminist framework. Sarah founded Body Stories (bodystories. nyc), an oral narrative project collecting and sharing stories about body experience. Sarah is interested in the intersection of personal and public dialogues around health, weight, beauty and identity.

Lauren Mitchell is one of the founders of The Doula Project. She received her M.S. from Columbia University's Program in Narrative Medicine in 2012, while working as a full-spectrum doula and as co-coordinator of the Reproductive Choices service at New York City hospital. She has worked with over a thousand clients throughout the spectrum of choice and trained hundreds of medical students, activists, as well as healthcare providers in methods of narrative-based compassionate care. She is currently a doctoral candidate in the Department of English at Vanderbilt University, where years of hands-on clinical experience inform her research.

Christine H. Morton, PhD, is a medical sociologist whose research and publications have focused on women's reproductive experiences and maternity care advocacy roles, including the doula and childbirth educator. In 1998, she founded an online listserve for social scientists studying reproduction, ReproNetwork.org. Since 2008, she has been at Stanford University's California Maternal Quality Care Collaborative. She is the author of *Birth Ambassadors: Doulas and the Re-emergence of Woman-Supported Birth in the United States* (Praeclarus Press, 2014).

Annie Robinson, MS, received a master's in Narrative Medicine at Columbia University. She is a coordinator of The Doula Project in New York City, and provides compassionate care for individuals across the spectrum of pregnancy. As a writer and teacher, Annie helps people explore the healing potential of interweaving stories, spirituality, and somatic experience.

Marla Seacrist, RN, PhD, is a tenured faculty member at California State University Stanislaus and is a practising labour and delivery nurse, and has worked with women during birth for twenty-nine years. Her research interests include labour and delivery nurse attitudes toward termination of pregnancy, perinatal bereavement, and maternal mortality.

Julie Johnson Searcy, MA, ABD, is a PhD candidate in anthropology and communication and culture at Indiana University. Her dissertation research in South Africa examines the space where reproduction, disease and technology intersect as women navigate pregnancy, birth, and high rates of HIV/AIDS infection. Interested in issues of gender, reproduction and performance, she also works as a doula and childbirth educator.

Vania Smith-Oka is an associate professor of anthropology at the University of Notre Dame, U.S. Her work addresses issues of marginality, reproduction, maternity, and motherhood in Mexico. She has carried out research among rural indigenous women navigating a large-scale development program as well as the complex interactions between clinicians and low-income women in an urban public hospital. She is the author of *Shaping the Motherhood of Indigenous Mexico* (Vanderbilt University Press, 2013).

Susanna C. Snyder, MA, is a medical anthropologist and the women's health policy specialist at the Colorado Department of Health Care Policy and Financing. Her graduate research with marginalized populations of pregnant women, including women placing children for adoption, prepared her for her current position where she manages and evaluates Medicaid programs for high-risk pregnant and parenting women. Susanna is also a doula and board member for The Family Room Access, a nonprofit that provides free and low-cost childbirth and parenting classes to low-income families.

Jennifer M. C. Torres is a research scientist at Michigan Public Health Institute, where she conducts research on maternal child health and tribal health and wellness. She received her PhD in sociology from University of Michigan in 2014. Her dissertation, conducted in the Midwest U.S., is an ethnographic study of doulas, lactation consultants, and their roles within the medical maternity system.